METABOLIC CONFUSION DIET COOKBOOK

New Edition Guide for Weight Loss & Optimal Health with Tasty Recipes for Breakfast, Lunch, Dinner, & Dessert, for Every Age & Lifestyle Including 30-Day Meal Plan.

Andrew H. Steve

About the Author

Andrew H. Steve, a renowned nutrition and health expert, specializes in empowering individuals over 40 to reclaim their health. With a passion for nutrition and a deep understanding of the human body and metabolism, Andrew has successfully guided many to achieve significant weight loss and enhanced well-being.

With over a decade of experience, Andrew's approach is far from one-size-fits-all. He tailors his advice to each individual, focusing on a holistic method that encompasses a balanced diet, mindful eating, and an active lifestyle, rather than just diets and restrictions.

Known for his ability to distill complex dietary concepts into practical, actionable strategies, Andrew is a guiding force in navigating the intricacies of metabolism and wellness. His dedication extends beyond his professional achievements, as he finds joy in outdoor activities, experimenting with new recipes, and engaging in healthy discussions.

If you're over 40 and looking to lose weight, increase energy, or improve your overall well-being, Andrew H. Steve is your ideal mentor. Under his guidance, you're not just adopting a healthy lifestyle; you're embarking on a transformative journey to rediscover your vitality and thrive.

TABLE OF CONTENTS

INTRODUCTION

In the bustling world we inhabit, where time is a precious commodity and the demands of modern life seem ceaseless, our relationship with food often becomes an afterthought—a hurried meal squeezed between meetings, a quick fix to quell hunger pangs, or an indulgence to soothe the stresses of the day. Amidst this whirlwind of activity, it's no wonder that many of us find ourselves feeling disconnected from our bodies, yearning for a sense of balance, vitality, and renewed energy.

If you're reading this, chances are you've experienced the frustration of trying countless diets, only to be met with fleeting results and a lingering sense of disappointment. Perhaps you've felt the pang of guilt after succumbing to yet another midnight snack, or the nagging voice of self-doubt as you stand before the mirror, wishing for a healthier, happier version of yourself. Know that you are not alone. In a world inundated with conflicting nutrition advice and fad diets promising quick fixes, it's easy to feel overwhelmed and disillusioned.

But fear not, for within the pages of this cookbook lies a beacon of hope—a guiding light illuminating the path to a healthier, more vibrant you. Welcome to the Metabolic Confusion Diet Cookbook, where we invite you to embark on a journey of culinary exploration, self-discovery, and transformation. More than just a collection of recipes, this cookbook is a testament to the power of mindful eating, nourishing your body from the inside out, and reclaiming your health and vitality.

So, what exactly is the Metabolic Confusion Diet, you might ask? At its core, it's a holistic approach to nutrition that harnesses the principles of metabolic confusion—a concept rooted in the idea of keeping your body guessing, preventing adaptation, and ultimately revving up your metabolism for optimal fat loss and sustained energy levels. Unlike traditional diets that rely on strict calorie counting or rigid meal plans, the Metabolic Confusion Diet celebrates variety, flexibility, and above all, enjoyment in the culinary experience.

Here, you won't find lists of forbidden foods or draconian rules dictating every morsel that passes your lips. Instead, we invite you to embrace the rich tapestry of flavors, textures, and ingredients that nature has to offer—exploring new tastes, experimenting with bold combinations, and savoring each bite with intention and gratitude. Whether you're a seasoned chef or a novice in the kitchen, our recipes are designed to inspire creativity, ignite your passion for cooking, and awaken your senses to the infinite possibilities of wholesome, nourishing cuisine.

But perhaps the most transformative aspect of the Metabolic Confusion Diet lies not in the meals themselves, but in the profound shift it inspires in our relationship with food. Gone are the days of viewing eating as a mere act of sustenance—a chore to be completed amidst the chaos of our daily lives. Instead, we invite you to cultivate a deeper awareness of the foods you consume, listening to the subtle cues of your body, and honoring its innate wisdom to guide you towards greater health and vitality.

As you journey through the pages of this cookbook, you'll discover a treasure trove of mouthwatering recipes—from hearty breakfasts to satisfying lunches, flavorful dinners to decadent desserts—all carefully crafted to nourish your body, tantalize your taste buds, and ignite your passion for wholesome, delicious cuisine. But beyond the recipes themselves, you'll find practical tips, insightful advice, and gentle encouragement to support you every step of the way.

Whether you're looking to shed a few pounds, boost your energy levels, or simply cultivate a healthier relationship with food, the Metabolic Confusion Diet Cookbook offers a roadmap to achieving your wellness goals—one delicious meal at a time. So, let go of the notion of dieting as deprivation, and embrace it as a celebration of abundance—a joyful journey towards a healthier, happier you.

In the pages that follow, we invite you to embark on a culinary adventure unlike any other—a journey of self-discovery, empowerment, and transformation. Together, let's unlock the full potential of our bodies, nourishing them with love, intention, and the nourishing power of delicious, wholesome cuisine. The path to vibrant health and vitality awaits—let's embark on this journey together.

CHAPTER 1

Metabolic Confusion stands as a revolutionary approach to weight management and overall health. In this chapter, we delve into the fundamental concepts behind Metabolic Confusion, exploring its definition, its impact on weight loss, and the numerous benefits it offers to those seeking a healthier lifestyle.

What is Metabolic Confusion?

Metabolic Confusion is a dietary strategy grounded in the principle of constantly varying calorie intake, macronutrient composition, and meal timing. The core idea behind Metabolic Confusion is to prevent the body from adapting to a fixed pattern of eating, which could lead to metabolic slowdown and weight loss plateaus.

At its essence, Metabolic Confusion mimics the natural fluctuations in food availability that our ancestors experienced. Our bodies are adept at adapting to routine, which is why traditional diets often lose their effectiveness over time. By introducing variability in our eating patterns, we keep our metabolism guessing, thereby maximizing calorie burning and fat loss.

This approach involves rotating between high-calorie and low-calorie days, altering macronutrient ratios, and occasionally incorporating periods of fasting. By constantly changing the nutritional stimuli we provide to our bodies, we stimulate metabolic flexibility and optimize fat-burning mechanisms.

Metabolic Confusion isn't just about what you eat; it's also about when you eat. Intermittent fasting, for example, is a common practice within the Metabolic Confusion framework. By incorporating periods of fasting, we give our digestive system a break, allowing our bodies to tap into stored fat for energy.

How Metabolic Confusion Affects Weight Loss

The traditional approach to weight loss often involves drastic calorie restriction and monotonous meal plans. While this may yield initial results, the body quickly adapts to the reduced calorie intake by slowing down metabolism and conserving energy. This adaptive response can stall progress and make further weight loss increasingly challenging.

Metabolic Confusion, on the other hand, disrupts this cycle of adaptation by constantly varying dietary inputs. By cycling between high-calorie and low-calorie days, we prevent our metabolism from settling into a predictable pattern. This constant state of flux keeps our metabolic rate elevated, allowing for more efficient calorie burning and fat loss.

Moreover, Metabolic Confusion promotes metabolic flexibility, which refers to the body's ability to switch between different fuel sources, such as glucose and fat. By incorporating periods of fasting and altering macronutrient ratios, we train our bodies to become more adept at utilizing stored fat for energy, thereby accelerating the fat loss process.

Another key aspect of Metabolic Confusion is its impact on hormone regulation. Traditional dieting can disrupt hormonal balance, leading to increased hunger, cravings, and metabolic slowdown. In contrast, Metabolic Confusion helps regulate hormones such as insulin, leptin, and ghrelin, which play crucial roles in appetite control and energy balance.

Furthermore, the psychological benefits of Metabolic Confusion cannot be overstated. Traditional diets often impose strict rules and restrictions, which can lead to feelings of deprivation and guilt. In contrast, Metabolic Confusion allows for greater flexibility and enjoyment in eating, making it easier to adhere to in the long term.

In summary, Metabolic Confusion represents a paradigm shift in the way we approach weight loss. By harnessing the power of variability and flexibility, we can overcome the body's natural tendency to adapt and plateau, achieving sustainable results that promote not only weight loss but also overall health and well-being.

Benefits of the Metabolic Confusion Diet

The Metabolic Confusion Diet offers a myriad of benefits beyond just weight loss. Here are some of the key advantages:

1. **Increased Metabolic Rate:** By constantly varying calorie intake and meal timing, Metabolic Confusion keeps the body's metabolic rate elevated, leading to more efficient calorie burning and fat loss.

2. **Improved Insulin Sensitivity:** Metabolic Confusion helps regulate blood sugar levels and improve insulin sensitivity, reducing the risk of type 2 diabetes and metabolic syndrome.

3. **Enhanced Fat-Burning Mechanisms:** By promoting metabolic flexibility and hormone regulation, Metabolic Confusion helps the body become more efficient at utilizing stored fat for energy, leading to accelerated fat loss.

4. **Greater Dietary Flexibility:** Unlike traditional diets that impose rigid meal plans and restrictions, Metabolic Confusion allows for greater flexibility in food choices and eating patterns, making it easier to adhere to in the long term.

5. **Reduced Risk of Plateaus:** Traditional diets often lead to weight loss plateaus as the body adapts to reduced calorie intake. Metabolic Confusion prevents plateaus by constantly varying dietary inputs, ensuring continued progress towards weight loss goals.

6. **Improved Mental Well-being:** The flexible nature of the Metabolic Confusion Diet promotes a positive relationship with food and reduces feelings of deprivation and guilt commonly associated with traditional dieting.

7. **Long-Term Sustainability:** Perhaps the most significant benefit of the Metabolic Confusion Diet is its long-term sustainability. By incorporating principles of variability and flexibility, Metabolic Confusion offers a sustainable approach to weight management and overall health.

CHAPTER 2

GETTING STARTED WITH THE METABOLIC CONFUSION DIET

Assessing Your Current Eating Habits

Assessing your current eating habits is the crucial first step towards embarking on the Metabolic Confusion Diet journey. It involves introspection, observation, and a willingness to confront your dietary patterns head-on.

Begin by keeping a food journal for at least a week. Document everything you eat and drink throughout the day, including portion sizes and any snacks or beverages consumed between meals. Be honest and detailed in your recordings, as this will provide valuable insights into your eating habits.

As you review your food journal, pay attention to patterns and trends. Are you consuming more processed foods than whole foods? Do you tend to overeat during certain times of the day or in specific situations? Are there emotional triggers that prompt you to eat even when you're not hungry?

Next, evaluate the nutritional content of your diet. Are you getting enough fruits and vegetables? Are you consuming an excessive amount of sugar, salt, or unhealthy fats? Assessing the balance of macronutrients (carbohydrates, proteins, and fats) in your meals can also help identify areas for improvement.

Consider your eating environment as well. Do you often eat on the go or in front of the television? Are mealtimes rushed or irregular? These factors can influence your eating habits and digestion.

Once you have a clear understanding of your current eating habits, identify areas where you can make positive changes. Set realistic goals based on your findings, whether it's reducing your intake of sugary snacks, increasing your vegetable consumption, or establishing regular meal times.

The goal of assessing your current eating habits is not to judge or criticize yourself but to gain insight and create a roadmap for healthier choices. Embrace this process as a learning opportunity and a crucial step towards transforming your relationship with food.

Planning Your Meals for Success

Meal planning is a cornerstone of the Metabolic Confusion Diet, providing structure, organization, and accountability to your dietary goals. By thoughtfully preparing your meals in advance, you can optimize nutrition, save time and money, and reduce the temptation to make impulsive food choices.

Start by establishing a weekly meal planning routine. Choose a designated day each week to plan your meals, taking into account your schedule, preferences, and nutritional needs. Set aside time to browse recipes, create a shopping list, and prepare ingredients for the week ahead.

When planning your meals, aim for variety and balance. Incorporate a diverse range of fruits, vegetables, whole grains, lean proteins, and healthy fats to ensure you're meeting your nutritional requirements. Experiment with new recipes and flavors to keep meals exciting and satisfying.

Consider batch cooking and meal prepping as time-saving strategies. Cook large batches of staple foods such as grains, beans, and proteins, then portion them out into individual containers for easy grab-and-go meals throughout the week. Pre-cutting vegetables, washing fruits, and assembling snack packs can also streamline your meal preparation process.

Don't forget to factor in flexibility and spontaneity when planning your meals. Leave room for occasional indulgences or dining out experiences while staying mindful of your overall dietary goals. Be adaptable and willing to adjust your meal plan as needed based on changing circumstances or preferences.

Finally, involve your family or household members in the meal planning process whenever possible. Solicit their input, accommodate their dietary preferences, and encourage their participation in grocery shopping and meal preparation activities. Making mealtime a collaborative and enjoyable experience can foster a sense of unity and shared responsibility for health and wellness.

By embracing meal planning as a proactive approach to nourishment and self-care, you can set yourself up for success on the Metabolic Confusion Diet and beyond.

Grocery Shopping Guide for the Metabolic Confusion Diet

Navigating the grocery store can be overwhelming, especially when trying to adhere to a specific dietary plan like the Metabolic Confusion Diet. However, with careful planning and strategic shopping strategies, you can confidently select nutritious foods that align with your health goals.

Before heading to the grocery store, take inventory of your pantry, refrigerator, and freezer. Dispose of any expired or unhealthy items, and make note of staple ingredients that need replenishing. Having a clear understanding of what you already have on hand will prevent duplicate purchases and ensure you're making efficient use of your shopping trip.

Create a detailed shopping list based on your meal plan for the week. Organize your list by food categories (e.g., produce, dairy, protein, pantry staples) to streamline your shopping experience and minimize backtracking through the store. Include specific quantities and ingredients to prevent overspending and reduce food waste.

When selecting fresh produce, prioritize seasonal and locally grown options whenever possible. Choose a variety of colorful fruits and vegetables to maximize nutrient intake and flavor diversity. Opt for organic or pesticide-free produce if available and within your budget.

In the protein aisle, focus on lean sources such as poultry, fish, tofu, legumes, and eggs. Look for grass-fed or pasture-raised meat and poultry, wild-caught fish, and organic or free-range eggs whenever feasible. Consider plant-based protein alternatives as well, including lentils, chickpeas, quinoa, and tempeh.

When perusing the aisles for grains and carbohydrates, opt for whole grains and complex carbohydrates over refined and processed options. Choose brown rice, quinoa, whole wheat pasta, oats, and barley for sustained energy and fiber content. Explore alternative grain varieties such as farro, bulgur, and millet to add variety to your meals.

Be discerning when selecting packaged and processed foods, carefully reading labels for hidden sugars, additives, and preservatives. Choose minimally processed options with recognizable ingredients lists and limited added sugars and sodium. Compare nutritional labels and opt for products with lower calorie, fat, and sodium content whenever possible.

Don't forget about hydration! Stock up on plenty of water, herbal teas, and other low-calorie beverages to stay hydrated throughout the day. Limit sugary sodas, energy drinks, and fruit juices, which can contribute to excess calorie consumption and disrupt metabolic balance.

Finally, practice mindful shopping by avoiding impulse purchases and sticking to your predetermined shopping list. Be open to trying new foods and incorporating seasonal ingredients into your meals. With careful planning and informed decision-making, you can navigate the grocery store with confidence and support your Metabolic Confusion Diet goals effectively.

CHAPTER 3

BREAKFAST RECIPES

1. Berry Blast Smoothie

Prep Time: 5 minutes
Serving Size: 1

Ingredients:

- ½ cup mixed berries (strawberries, blueberries, raspberries)
- ½ banana
- ½ cup spinach leaves
- ½ cup unsweetened almond milk
- ¼ cup Greek yogurt
- 1 tablespoon chia seeds
- Ice cubes (optional)

Instructions:

1. Combine all ingredients in a blender.
2. Blend until smooth and creamy.
3. Add ice cubes if desired for a colder texture.
4. Pour into a glass and serve immediately.

Nutritional Information:

- Calories: 250
- Protein: 10g

- Carbohydrates: 35g

- Fat: 8g

- Fiber: 9g

2. Veggie Egg Muffins

Prep Time: 10 minutes
Cooking Time: 20 minutes
Serving Size: 2 muffins

Ingredients:

- 4 eggs

- ¼ cup diced bell peppers

- ¼ cup diced tomatoes

- ¼ cup chopped spinach

- 2 tablespoons diced onions

- Salt and pepper to taste

- Cooking spray

Instructions:

1. Preheat the oven to 350°F (175°C). Grease a muffin tin with cooking spray.

2. In a mixing bowl, whisk the eggs until well beaten.

3. Stir in the diced vegetables and season with salt and pepper.

4. Pour the egg mixture evenly into the muffin tin, filling each cup about 3/4 full.

5. Bake in the preheated oven for 20 minutes or until the egg muffins are set and slightly golden on top.

6. Allow the egg muffins to cool slightly before removing them from the muffin tin.

7. Serve warm or refrigerate for later consumption.

Nutritional Information:

- Calories: 120 per serving

- Protein: 10g

- Carbohydrates: 5g

- Fat: 7g

- Fiber: 1g

3. Avocado Toast

Prep Time: 5 minutes
Cooking Time: 5 minutes
Serving Size: 1

Ingredients:

- 1 slice whole grain bread

- ½ ripe avocado

- ½ teaspoon lemon juice

- Pinch of red pepper flakes (optional)

- Salt and pepper to taste

Instructions:

1. Toast the whole grain bread until golden brown.

2. In a small bowl, mash the ripe avocado with lemon juice, red pepper flakes (if using), salt, and pepper.

3. Spread the mashed avocado evenly onto the toasted bread.

4. Garnish with additional toppings like sliced tomatoes, radishes, or microgreens if desired.

5. Serve immediately.

Nutritional Information:

- Calories: 200

- Protein: 5g

- Carbohydrates: 15g

- Fat: 12g

- Fiber: 6g

4. Greek Yogurt Parfait

Prep Time: 5 minutes
Serving Size: 1

Ingredients:

- ½ cup Greek yogurt

- ¼ cup granola (choose low-sugar options)

- ¼ cup mixed berries (strawberries, blueberries, raspberries)

- 1 tablespoon honey (optional)

Instructions:

1. In a serving glass or bowl, layer Greek yogurt, granola, and mixed berries.

2. Repeat the layers until the glass or bowl is filled.

3. Drizzle honey on top if desired for added sweetness.

4. Serve immediately as a nutritious and satisfying breakfast option.

Nutritional Information:

- Calories: 250

- Protein: 15g

- Carbohydrates: 35g

- Fat: 6g

- Fiber: 5g

5. Spinach and Mushroom Omelette

Prep Time: 10 minutes
Cooking Time: 10 minutes
Serving Size: 1

Ingredients:

- 2 eggs

- ¼ cup chopped spinach

- ¼ cup sliced mushrooms

- 2 tablespoons diced onions

- 1 tablespoon olive oil

- Salt and pepper to taste

Instructions:

1. In a small bowl, whisk the eggs until well beaten. Season with salt and pepper.

2. Heat olive oil in a non-stick skillet over medium heat.

3. Add diced onions and sliced mushrooms to the skillet. Sauté until softened.

4. Add chopped spinach to the skillet and cook until wilted.

5. Pour the beaten eggs over the vegetables, spreading them evenly across the skillet.

6. Cook until the eggs are set and the bottom is lightly golden brown.

7. Using a spatula, fold the omelette in half and transfer it to a plate.

8. Serve hot with a side of whole grain toast or fresh fruit.

Nutritional Information:

- Calories: 220

- Protein: 14g

- Carbohydrates: 5g

- Fat: 16g

- Fiber: 2g

6. Quinoa Breakfast Bowl

Prep Time: 10 minutes
Cooking Time: 15 minutes
Serving Size: 1

Ingredients:

- ½ cup cooked quinoa
- ¼ cup sliced strawberries
- ¼ cup sliced bananas
- 2 tablespoons chopped almonds
- 1 tablespoon honey
- ¼ teaspoon cinnamon

Instructions:

1. In a serving bowl, layer cooked quinoa, sliced strawberries, sliced bananas, and chopped almonds.

2. Drizzle honey over the top and sprinkle with cinnamon.

3. Stir gently to combine all ingredients.

4. Serve warm or cold as a nutritious and filling breakfast option.

Nutritional Information:

- Calories: 300
- Protein: 8g
- Carbohydrates: 45g

- Fat: 10g

- Fiber: 6g

7. Chia Seed Pudding

Prep Time: 5 minutes (plus chilling time)
Serving Size: 1

Ingredients:

- 2 tablespoons chia seeds

- ½ cup unsweetened almond milk

- ¼ teaspoon vanilla extract

- 1 teaspoon honey or maple syrup (optional)

- Sliced fruit for garnish (e.g., strawberries, kiwi, mango)

Instructions:

1. In a small bowl or jar, combine chia seeds, almond milk, vanilla extract, and honey or maple syrup (if using).

2. Stir well to combine all ingredients.

3. Cover the bowl or jar and refrigerate for at least 2 hours or overnight to allow the chia seeds to absorb the liquid and thicken.

4. Once chilled and thickened, stir the chia seed pudding again to ensure even consistency.

5. Serve in a bowl or glass, topped with sliced fruit for added flavour and texture.

6. Enjoy as a nutritious and satisfying breakfast or snack option.

Nutritional Information:

- Calories: 180

- Protein: 5g

- Carbohydrates: 20g

- Fat: 9g

- Fiber: 10g

8. Peanut Butter Banana Smoothie

Prep Time: 5 minutes
Serving Size: 1

Ingredients:

- 1 ripe banana

- 1 tablespoon peanut butter

- ½ cup unsweetened almond milk

- ¼ cup Greek yogurt

- ¼ teaspoon vanilla extract

- Ice cubes (optional)

Instructions:

1. In a blender, combine the ripe banana, peanut butter, almond milk, Greek yogurt, and vanilla extract.

2. Blend until smooth and creamy.

3. Add ice cubes if desired for a colder texture.

4. Pour into a glass and serve immediately as a delicious and protein-rich breakfast option.

Nutritional Information:

- Calories: 280

- Protein: 10g

- Carbohydrates: 30g

- Fat: 14g

- Fiber: 6g

9. Blueberry Oatmeal

Prep Time: 5 minutes
Cooking Time: 10 minutes
Serving Size: 1

Ingredients:

- ½ cup rolled oats

- 1 cup water or unsweetened almond milk

- ¼ cup fresh or frozen blueberries

- 1 tablespoon honey or maple syrup

- Pinch of cinnamon

- Chopped nuts or seeds for garnish (optional)

Instructions:

1. In a small saucepan, combine rolled oats and water or almond milk.

2. Bring to a boil, then reduce heat and simmer for 5-7 minutes, stirring occasionally, until the oats are cooked and the mixture has thickened.

3. Stir in fresh or frozen blueberries, honey or maple syrup, and a pinch of cinnamon.

4. Continue to cook for an additional 2-3 minutes until the blueberries are heated through and the oatmeal is creamy.

5. Remove from heat and transfer to a serving bowl.

6. Garnish with chopped nuts or seeds if desired.

7. Serve hot and enjoy a warm and comforting breakfast option.

Nutritional Information:

- Calories: 300

- Protein: 8g

- Carbohydrates: 50g

- Fat: 6g

- Fiber: 8g

10. Veggie Breakfast Burrito

Prep Time: 10 minutes
Cooking Time: 10 minutes
Serving Size: 1

Ingredients:

- 1 whole grain tortilla
- 2 eggs, scrambled
- ¼ cup diced bell peppers
- ¼ cup diced tomatoes
- 2 tablespoons diced onions
- ¼ avocado, sliced
- Salsa or hot sauce for serving (optional)

Instructions:

1. In a non-stick skillet, scramble the eggs until cooked through. Set aside.

2. In the same skillet, sauté diced bell peppers, diced tomatoes, and diced onions until softened.

3. Warm the whole grain tortilla in the skillet or microwave for a few seconds to make it pliable.

4. Place the scrambled eggs and sautéed vegetables in the centre of the tortilla.

5. Top with sliced avocado and a drizzle of salsa or hot sauce if desired.

6. Fold the sides of the tortilla over the filling to create a burrito shape.

7. Serve immediately as a hearty and satisfying breakfast option.

Nutritional Information:

- Calories: 350
- Protein: 15g
- Carbohydrates: 35g
- Fat: 15g
- Fiber: 8g

11. Overnight Oats

Prep Time: 5 minutes (plus chilling time)
Serving Size: 1

Ingredients:

- ½ cup rolled oats
- ½ cup unsweetened almond milk
- ¼ cup Greek yogurt
- 1 tablespoon chia seeds
- 1 tablespoon honey or maple syrup
- ¼ teaspoon vanilla extract
- Sliced fruit for garnish (e.g., bananas, strawberries, kiwi)

Instructions:

1. In a mason jar or bowl, combine rolled oats, almond milk, Greek yogurt, chia seeds, honey or maple syrup, and vanilla extract.
2. Stir well to combine all ingredients.

3. Cover the jar or bowl and refrigerate overnight or for at least 4 hours to allow the oats to absorb the liquid and soften.

4. Once chilled and thickened, stir the overnight oats again to ensure even consistency.

5. Top with sliced fruit before serving for added flavour and texture.

6. Enjoy cold as a convenient and nutritious breakfast option.

Nutritional Information:

- Calories: 300

- Protein: 12g

- Carbohydrates: 45g

- Fat: 8g

- Fiber: 10g

12. Sweet Potato Breakfast Hash

Prep Time: 10 minutes
Cooking Time: 20 minutes
Serving Size: 2

Ingredients:

- 2 medium sweet potatoes, peeled and diced

- ½ bell pepper, diced

- ½ onion, diced

- 2 cloves garlic, minced

- 2 tablespoons olive oil

- 1 teaspoon paprika

- ½ teaspoon cumin

- Salt and pepper to taste

- 2 eggs (optional, for serving)

Instructions:

1. Heat olive oil in a skillet over medium heat.

2. Add diced sweet potatoes to the skillet and cook for 8-10 minutes, stirring occasionally, until golden brown and tender.

3. Add diced bell pepper, diced onion, and minced garlic to the skillet. Sauté for an additional 5-7 minutes until the vegetables are softened.

4. Season the hash with paprika, cumin, salt, and pepper, stirring to combine.

5. If desired, create wells in the hash and crack eggs into each well.

6. Cover the skillet and cook for 5-7 minutes until the eggs are set to your liking.

7. Serve hot as a satisfying and flavourful breakfast option.

Nutritional Information:

- Calories: 250 per serving (without eggs)

- Protein: 5g

- Carbohydrates: 30g

- Fat: 12g

- Fiber: 6g

13. Breakfast Quinoa Bowl

Prep Time: 10 minutes
Cooking Time: 15 minutes
Serving Size: 1

Ingredients:

- ½ cup cooked quinoa

- ¼ cup sliced strawberries

- ¼ cup sliced bananas

- 2 tablespoons chopped almonds

- 1 tablespoon honey

- ¼ teaspoon cinnamon

Instructions:

1. In a serving bowl, layer cooked quinoa, sliced strawberries, sliced bananas, and chopped almonds.

2. Drizzle honey over the top and sprinkle with cinnamon.

3. Stir gently to combine all ingredients.

4. Serve warm or cold as a nutritious and filling breakfast option.

Nutritional Information:

- Calories: 300
- Protein: 8g
- Carbohydrates: 45g
- Fat: 10g
- Fiber: 6g

14. Banana Nut Overnight Oats

Prep Time: 5 minutes (plus chilling time)
Serving Size: 1

Ingredients:

- ½ cup rolled oats
- ½ cup unsweetened almond milk
- ½ ripe banana, mashed
- 1 tablespoon chopped walnuts
- 1 tablespoon honey or maple syrup
- ¼ teaspoon vanilla extract
- Pinch of cinnamon

Instructions:

1. In a mason jar or bowl, combine rolled oats, almond milk, mashed banana, chopped walnuts, honey or maple syrup, vanilla extract, and cinnamon.

2. Stir well to combine all ingredients.

3. Cover the jar or bowl and refrigerate overnight or for at least 4 hours to allow the oats to absorb the liquid and soften.

4. Once chilled and thickened, stir the overnight oats again to ensure even consistency.

5. Serve cold as a convenient and delicious breakfast option.

Nutritional Information:

- Calories: 320

- Protein: 10g

- Carbohydrates: 50g

- Fat: 10g

- Fiber: 7g

15. Spinach and Feta Breakfast Wrap

Prep Time: 10 minutes
Cooking Time: 5 minutes
Serving Size: 1

Ingredients:

- 1 whole grain tortilla

- 2 eggs, scrambled

- ¼ cup chopped spinach

- 2 tablespoons crumbled feta cheese

- Salt and pepper to taste

Instructions:

1. In a non-stick skillet, scramble the eggs until cooked through. Set aside.

2. Warm the whole grain tortilla in the skillet or microwave for a few seconds to make it pliable.

3. Place the scrambled eggs, chopped spinach, and crumbled feta cheese in the centre of the tortilla.

4. Season with salt and pepper to taste.

5. Fold the sides of the tortilla over the filling to create a wrap.

6. Serve immediately as a flavourful and protein-rich breakfast option.

Nutritional Information:

- Calories: 320

- Protein: 15g

- Carbohydrates: 25g

- Fat: 18g

- Fiber: 5g

16. Mediterranean Breakfast Bowl

Prep Time: 10 minutes
Cooking Time: 15 minutes
Serving Size: 1

Ingredients:

- ½ cup cooked quinoa
- ¼ cup cherry tomatoes, halved
- 2 tablespoons chopped cucumber
- 2 tablespoons crumbled feta cheese
- 2 tablespoons kalamata olives, sliced
- 1 tablespoon chopped fresh parsley
- 1 tablespoon olive oil
- ½ tablespoon lemon juice
- Salt and pepper to taste

Instructions:

1. In a serving bowl, layer cooked quinoa, cherry tomatoes, chopped cucumber, crumbled feta cheese, and sliced kalamata olives.

2. Sprinkle chopped fresh parsley over the top.

3. In a small bowl, whisk together olive oil, lemon juice, salt, and pepper to make the dressing.

4. Drizzle the dressing over the breakfast bowl.

5. Serve immediately as a flavourful and nutrient-rich breakfast option.

Nutritional Information:

- Calories: 350
- Protein: 10g

- Carbohydrates: 35g

- Fat: 18g

- Fiber: 5g

17. Apple Cinnamon Overnight Oats

Prep Time: 5 minutes (plus chilling time)
Serving Size: 1

Ingredients:

- ½ cup rolled oats

- ½ cup unsweetened almond milk

- ½ apple, diced

- 1 tablespoon chopped almonds

- 1 tablespoon honey or maple syrup

- ¼ teaspoon cinnamon

- Pinch of nutmeg

Instructions:

1. In a mason jar or bowl, combine rolled oats, almond milk, diced apple, chopped almonds, honey or maple syrup, cinnamon, and nutmeg.

2. Stir well to combine all ingredients.

3. Cover the jar or bowl and refrigerate overnight or for at least 4 hours to allow the oats to absorb the liquid and soften.

4. Once chilled and thickened, stir the overnight oats again to ensure even consistency.

5. Serve cold as a delicious and filling breakfast option.

Nutritional Information:

- Calories: 330
- Protein: 9g
- Carbohydrates: 50g
- Fat: 12g
- Fiber: 8g

18. Banana Pancakes

Prep Time: 10 minutes
Cooking Time: 10 minutes
Serving Size: 2-3 pancakes

Ingredients:

- 1 ripe banana
- 2 eggs
- ¼ cup rolled oats
- ¼ teaspoon cinnamon
- Cooking spray or coconut oil for greasing the skillet
- Sliced fruit for serving (e.g., berries, bananas)

Instructions:

1. In a blender, combine ripe banana, eggs, rolled oats, and cinnamon. Blend until smooth and creamy.

2. Heat a non-stick skillet over medium heat and lightly grease with cooking spray or coconut oil.

3. Pour pancake batter onto the skillet, using about 1/4 cup for each pancake.

4. Cook for 2-3 minutes until bubbles form on the surface of the pancake.

5. Flip and cook for an additional 1-2 minutes until golden brown and cooked through.

6. Repeat with the remaining batter, greasing the skillet as needed.

7. Serve warm with sliced fruit for a nutritious and satisfying breakfast option.

Nutritional Information:

- Calories: 150 per pancake

- Protein: 6g

- Carbohydrates: 20g

- Fat: 5g

- Fiber: 3g

19. Green Smoothie Bowl

Prep Time: 5 minutes
Serving Size: 1

Ingredients:

- ½ cup spinach leaves

- ½ ripe avocado

- ½ cup frozen mango chunks

- ½ cup unsweetened almond milk

- 1 tablespoon chia seeds

- Sliced fruit and nuts for garnish (e.g., kiwi, almonds)

Instructions:

1. In a blender, combine spinach leaves, ripe avocado, frozen mango chunks, almond milk, and chia seeds.

2. Blend until smooth and creamy.

3. Pour the green smoothie into a serving bowl.

4. Top with sliced fruit and nuts for added texture and flavour.

5. Serve immediately as a nutrient-packed breakfast option.

Nutritional Information:

- Calories: 300

- Protein: 8g

- Carbohydrates: 30g

- Fat: 15g

- Fiber: 10g

20. Smoked Salmon and Cream Cheese Bagel

Prep Time: 5 minutes
Cooking Time: 5 minutes
Serving Size: 1

Ingredients:

- 1 whole grain bagel, sliced and toasted
- 2 tablespoons cream cheese
- 2 slices smoked salmon
- 1 tablespoon capers
- Fresh dill for garnish

Instructions:

1. Spread cream cheese evenly on each half of the toasted whole grain bagel.
2. Top one half of the bagel with smoked salmon slices.
3. Sprinkle capers over the smoked salmon.
4. Garnish with fresh dill for added flavour.
5. Sandwich the two halves of the bagel together.
6. Serve immediately as a delicious and protein-rich breakfast option.

Nutritional Information:

- Calories: 350
- Protein: 15g
- Carbohydrates: 35g
- Fat: 15g
- Fiber: 6g

CHAPTER 4

LUNCH RECIPES

1. Quinoa and Black Bean Salad

Prep Time: 15 minutes
Cooking Time: 15 minutes
Serving Size: 4

Ingredients:

- 1 cup quinoa, rinsed

- 2 cups water or vegetable broth

- 1 can (15 oz) black beans, drained and rinsed

- 1 red bell pepper, diced

- 1 cucumber, diced

- ¼ cup red onion, finely chopped

- ¼ cup fresh cilantro, chopped

- Juice of 1 lime

- 2 tablespoons olive oil

- Salt and pepper to taste

Instructions:

1. In a medium saucepan, bring the water or vegetable broth to a boil. Add the quinoa, reduce heat to low, cover, and simmer for 15 minutes or until all the liquid is absorbed.

2. Fluff the quinoa with a fork and transfer it to a large mixing bowl. Let it cool for a few minutes.

3. Add the black beans, red bell pepper, cucumber, red onion, and cilantro to the bowl with the quinoa.

4. In a small bowl, whisk together the lime juice, olive oil, salt, and pepper. Pour the dressing over the salad and toss gently to combine.

5. Serve chilled or at room temperature. Enjoy!

Nutritional Information per Serving:

- Calories: 320

- Protein: 12g

- Carbohydrates: 50g

- Fat: 9g

- Fiber: 10g

2. Grilled Chicken and Vegetable Skewers

Prep Time: 20 minutes
Cooking Time: 10 minutes
Serving Size: 4

Ingredients:

- 2 boneless, skinless chicken breasts, cut into cubes

- 1 zucchini, sliced

- 1 yellow bell pepper, cut into chunks

- 1 red onion, cut into chunks

- 8 cherry tomatoes

- 2 tablespoons olive oil

- 2 cloves garlic, minced

- Juice of 1 lemon

- 1 teaspoon dried oregano

- Salt and pepper to taste

Instructions:

1. In a bowl, combine the olive oil, minced garlic, lemon juice, dried oregano, salt, and pepper. Mix well to make the marinade.

2. Thread the chicken cubes and vegetables onto skewers, alternating between chicken and vegetables.

3. Place the skewers in a shallow dish and pour the marinade over them, making sure they are evenly coated. Let them marinate for at least 15 minutes.

4. Preheat the grill or grill pan over medium-high heat. Cook the skewers for about 4-5 minutes on each side or until the chicken is cooked through and the vegetables are tender.

5. Remove the skewers from the grill and serve hot. Enjoy with a side of brown rice or quinoa if desired.

Nutritional Information per Serving:

- Calories: 250

- Protein: 25g

- Carbohydrates: 10g

- Fat: 12g

- Fiber: 3g

3. Mediterranean Chickpea Salad

Prep Time: 15 minutes
Cooking Time: 0 minutes
Serving Size: 4

Ingredients:

- 2 cans (15 oz each) chickpeas, drained and rinsed

- 1 English cucumber, diced

- 1 cup cherry tomatoes, halved

- ½ red onion, thinly sliced

- ¼ cup Kalamata olives, pitted and sliced

- ¼ cup fresh parsley, chopped

- ¼ cup feta cheese, crumbled (optional)

- Juice of 1 lemon

- 2 tablespoons extra virgin olive oil

- 1 teaspoon dried oregano

- Salt and pepper to taste

Instructions:

1. In a large mixing bowl, combine the chickpeas, cucumber, cherry tomatoes, red onion, olives, and parsley.

2. In a small bowl, whisk together the lemon juice, olive oil, dried oregano, salt, and pepper to make the dressing.

3. Pour the dressing over the salad ingredients and toss gently to coat everything evenly.

4. Sprinkle crumbled feta cheese over the top of the salad if desired.

5. Serve chilled or at room temperature. Enjoy as a light and refreshing lunch option!

Nutritional Information per Serving:

- Calories: 280

- Protein: 12g

- Carbohydrates: 35g

- Fat: 11g

- Fiber: 9g

4. Turkey and Avocado Wrap

Prep Time: 10 minutes
Cooking Time: 0 minutes
Serving Size: 2

Ingredients:

- 4 large whole wheat tortillas

- 8 slices of deli turkey

- 1 ripe avocado, sliced

- 1 cup baby spinach leaves

- ½ cup cherry tomatoes, halved

- ¼ cup Greek yogurt

- 1 tablespoon Dijon mustard

- Salt and pepper to taste

Instructions:

1. Lay out the tortillas on a clean surface. Spread Greek yogurt and Dijon mustard evenly over each tortilla.

2. Divide the turkey slices, avocado slices, baby spinach, and cherry tomatoes evenly among the tortillas.

3. Season with salt and pepper to taste.

4. Roll up each tortilla tightly, folding in the sides as you go to create a wrap.

5. Slice each wrap in half diagonally and serve immediately, or wrap in parchment paper for a portable lunch option.

Nutritional Information per Serving (1 wrap):

- Calories: 320

- Protein: 18g

- Carbohydrates: 28g

- Fat: 15g

- Fiber: 8g

5. Tuna Salad Lettuce Wraps

Prep Time: 10 minutes
Cooking Time: 0 minutes
Serving Size: 2

Ingredients:

- 2 cans (5 oz each) tuna, drained
- ¼ cup celery, finely diced
- ¼ cup red onion, finely diced
- 2 tablespoons Greek yogurt
- 1 tablespoon lemon juice
- 1 teaspoon Dijon mustard
- Salt and pepper to taste
- 4 large lettuce leaves (such as romaine or butter lettuce)
- Optional toppings: sliced tomatoes, avocado, cucumber

Instructions:

1. In a mixing bowl, combine the drained tuna, diced celery, diced red onion, Greek yogurt, lemon juice, Dijon mustard, salt, and pepper. Mix well until everything is evenly combined.

2. Lay out the lettuce leaves on a clean surface. Divide the tuna salad mixture evenly among the lettuce leaves.

3. Add optional toppings such as sliced tomatoes, avocado, or cucumber if desired.

4. Roll up each lettuce leaf, tucking in the sides to create a wrap.

5. Serve immediately, or wrap in parchment paper for a convenient on-the-go lunch.

Nutritional Information per Serving (2 lettuce wraps):

- Calories: 180

- Protein: 25g

- Carbohydrates: 6g

- Fat: 6g

- Fiber: 2g

6. Veggie Stir-Fry with Tofu

Prep Time: 15 minutes
Cooking Time: 15 minutes
Serving Size: 4

Ingredients:

- 14 oz extra firm tofu, drained and pressed

- 2 tablespoons soy sauce or tamari

- 1 tablespoon sesame oil

- 1 tablespoon olive oil

- 2 cloves garlic, minced

- 1 tablespoon fresh ginger, minced

- 1 red bell pepper, thinly sliced

- 1 yellow bell pepper, thinly sliced

- 1 cup broccoli florets

- 1 cup snap peas

- 1 carrot, julienned

- 2 green onions, thinly sliced

- Cooked brown rice or quinoa for serving

Instructions:

1. Cut the tofu into cubes and place them in a shallow dish. Drizzle with soy sauce or tamari and let marinate for at least 10 minutes.

2. In a large skillet or wok, heat olive oil over medium-high heat. Add the marinated tofu cubes and cook until golden brown on all sides, about 5-7 minutes. Remove tofu from skillet and set aside.

3. In the same skillet, add sesame oil, garlic, and ginger. Cook for 1 minute until fragrant.

4. Add sliced bell peppers, broccoli florets, snap peas, and julienned carrot to the skillet. Stir-fry for 5-7 minutes until vegetables are tender-crisp.

5. Return the cooked tofu to the skillet and toss everything together.

6. Garnish with sliced green onions and serve hot over cooked brown rice or quinoa.

Nutritional Information per Serving (without rice or quinoa):

- Calories: 220
- Protein: 15g
- Carbohydrates: 14g
- Fat: 12g
- Fiber: 5g

7. Greek Chicken Salad

Prep Time: 20 minutes
Cooking Time: 20 minutes
Serving Size: 4

Ingredients:

- 2 boneless, skinless chicken breasts
- 1 tablespoon olive oil
- 1 teaspoon dried oregano
- Salt and pepper to taste
- 4 cups mixed salad greens
- 1 cucumber, sliced
- 1 cup cherry tomatoes, halved
- ½ red onion, thinly sliced
- ¼ cup Kalamata olives, pitted
- ¼ cup crumbled feta cheese
- Juice of 1 lemon

- 2 tablespoons extra virgin olive oil

Instructions:

1. Preheat oven to 375°F (190°C). Rub the chicken breasts with olive oil, dried oregano, salt, and pepper. Place on a baking sheet and bake for 20 minutes or until cooked through. Let cool and slice thinly.

2. In a large mixing bowl, combine the salad greens, sliced cucumber, cherry tomatoes, red onion, and Kalamata olives.

3. In a small bowl, whisk together the lemon juice and extra virgin olive oil to make the dressing.

4. Drizzle the dressing over the salad and toss gently to coat.

5. Divide the salad mixture among serving plates and top with sliced chicken and crumbled feta cheese.

6. Serve immediately, and enjoy this fresh and flavourful Greek-inspired salad!

Nutritional Information per Serving:

- Calories: 280
- Protein: 25g
- Carbohydrates: 10g
- Fat: 15g
- Fiber: 4g

8. Lentil and Vegetable Soup

Prep Time: 15 minutes
Cooking Time: 40 minutes
Serving Size: 6

Ingredients:

- 1 cup dried green or brown lentils, rinsed and drained
- 6 cups vegetable broth
- 1 onion, diced
- 2 carrots, diced
- 2 celery stalks, diced
- 2 cloves garlic, minced
- 1 teaspoon dried thyme
- 1 teaspoon dried rosemary
- Salt and pepper to taste
- 2 cups baby spinach leaves
- Juice of 1 lemon
- Fresh parsley for garnish

Instructions:

1. In a large pot, combine the lentils, vegetable broth, diced onion, diced carrots, diced celery, minced garlic, dried thyme, and dried rosemary. Bring to a boil over medium-high heat.

2. Reduce heat to low, cover, and simmer for 30-40 minutes, or until the lentils and vegetables are tender.

3. Season with salt and pepper to taste.

4. Stir in the baby spinach leaves and lemon juice, and cook for an additional 2-3 minutes until the spinach is wilted.

5. Ladle the soup into bowls and garnish with fresh parsley before serving.

6. Enjoy this hearty and nutritious lentil and vegetable soup as a satisfying lunch option!

Nutritional Information per Serving:

- Calories: 220

- Protein: 15g

- Carbohydrates: 35g

- Fat: 2g

- Fiber: 12g

9. Shrimp and Avocado Salad

Prep Time: 15 minutes
Cooking Time: 5 minutes
Serving Size: 2

Ingredients:

- ½ lb medium shrimp, peeled and deveined

- 1 tablespoon olive oil

- 1 teaspoon smoked paprika

- Salt and pepper to taste

- 4 cups mixed salad greens

- 1 avocado, diced

- ½ cup cherry tomatoes, halved

- ¼ cup red onion, thinly sliced

- Juice of 1 lime

- 2 tablespoons extra virgin olive oil

- Fresh cilantro for garnish

Instructions:

1. In a large skillet, heat olive oil over medium heat. Season the shrimp with smoked paprika, salt, and pepper, then add them to the skillet.

2. Cook the shrimp for 2-3 minutes on each side, until pink and opaque. Remove from heat and let cool slightly.

3. In a large mixing bowl, combine the salad greens, diced avocado, halved cherry tomatoes, and sliced red onion.

4. In a small bowl, whisk together the lime juice and extra virgin olive oil to make the dressing.

5. Drizzle the dressing over the salad and toss gently to coat.

6. Divide the salad mixture among serving plates and top with cooked shrimp.

7. Garnish with fresh cilantro before serving. Enjoy this light and flavourful shrimp and avocado salad!

Nutritional Information per Serving:

- Calories: 320
- Protein: 20g
- Carbohydrates: 15g
- Fat: 20g
- Fiber: 10g

10. Caprese Quinoa Salad

Prep Time: 15 minutes
Cooking Time: 15 minutes
Serving Size: 4

Ingredients:

- 1 cup quinoa, rinsed
- 2 cups water or vegetable broth
- 2 cups cherry tomatoes, halved
- 1 cup fresh mozzarella balls, halved
- ¼ cup fresh basil leaves, chopped
- 2 tablespoons balsamic vinegar
- 2 tablespoons extra virgin olive oil
- Salt and pepper to taste

Instructions:

1. In a medium saucepan, bring the water or vegetable broth to a boil. Add the quinoa, reduce heat to low, cover, and simmer for 15 minutes or until all the liquid is absorbed.

2. Fluff the quinoa with a fork and transfer it to a large mixing bowl. Let it cool for a few minutes.

3. Add the cherry tomatoes, fresh mozzarella balls, and chopped basil leaves to the bowl with the quinoa.

4. In a small bowl, whisk together the balsamic vinegar, extra virgin olive oil, salt, and pepper. Pour the dressing over the salad and toss gently to combine.

5. Serve chilled or at room temperature. Enjoy this delightful Caprese quinoa salad as a light and satisfying lunch option!

Nutritional Information per Serving:

- Calories: 280
- Protein: 12g
- Carbohydrates: 35g
- Fat: 10g
- Fiber: 5g

11. Chicken and Vegetable Stir-Fry

Prep Time: 20 minutes
Cooking Time: 15 minutes
Serving Size: 4

Ingredients:

- 2 boneless, skinless chicken breasts, thinly sliced
- 2 tablespoons soy sauce or tamari
- 1 tablespoon cornstarch
- 2 tablespoons olive oil
- 2 cloves garlic, minced
- 1 tablespoon fresh ginger, minced
- 1 red bell pepper, thinly sliced
- 1 yellow bell pepper, thinly sliced
- 1 cup broccoli florets
- 1 cup snap peas
- 1 carrot, julienned
- 2 green onions, thinly sliced
- Cooked brown rice or quinoa for serving

Instructions:

1. In a bowl, combine the sliced chicken breast, soy sauce or tamari, and cornstarch. Mix well and let marinate for 10 minutes.

2. Heat olive oil in a large skillet or wok over medium-high heat. Add minced garlic and ginger, and cook for 1 minute until fragrant.

3. Add the marinated chicken slices to the skillet and stir-fry for 5-7 minutes until cooked through and golden brown. Remove from skillet and set aside.

4. In the same skillet, add the sliced bell peppers, broccoli florets, snap peas, and julienned carrot. Stir-fry for 5-7 minutes until vegetables are tender-crisp.

5. Return the cooked chicken to the skillet and toss everything together.

6. Garnish with sliced green onions and serve hot over cooked brown rice or quinoa.

Nutritional Information per Serving (without rice or quinoa):

- Calories: 280

- Protein: 25g

- Carbohydrates: 15g

- Fat: 12g

- Fiber: 5g

12. Spinach and Mushroom Quesadillas

Prep Time: 15 minutes
Cooking Time: 10 minutes
Serving Size: 4

Ingredients:

- 8 whole wheat tortillas

- 2 cups fresh spinach leaves

- 1 cup mushrooms, sliced

- ½ cup red bell pepper, diced

- ½ cup onion, diced

- 1 cup shredded cheese (cheddar, mozzarella, or a blend)

- 2 tablespoons olive oil

- Salt and pepper to taste

- Salsa and Greek yogurt for serving (optional)

Instructions:

1. Heat olive oil in a large skillet over medium heat. Add diced onion and cook until translucent, about 3-4 minutes.

2. Add sliced mushrooms and diced red bell pepper to the skillet. Cook until vegetables are tender, about 5 minutes.

3. Add fresh spinach leaves to the skillet and cook until wilted, about 2 minutes. Season with salt and pepper to taste.

4. Remove vegetables from the skillet and set aside. Wipe the skillet clean.

5. Place one tortilla in the skillet over medium heat. Sprinkle shredded cheese over the tortilla, then add a layer of cooked vegetables.

6. Top with another tortilla and cook until the bottom tortilla is golden brown and crispy, about 3-4 minutes.

7. Carefully flip the quesadilla and cook until the other side is golden brown and crispy, about 3-4 minutes more.

8. Repeat with remaining tortillas and filling ingredients.

9. Cut quesadillas into wedges and serve hot, with salsa and Greek yogurt on the side if desired.

Nutritional Information per Serving (1/4 of the recipe):

- Calories: 350

- Protein: 15g

- Carbohydrates: 35g

- Fat: 15g

- Fiber: 6g

13. Asian-Inspired Tofu Bowl

Prep Time: 20 minutes
Cooking Time: 15 minutes
Serving Size: 4

Ingredients:

- 14 oz extra firm tofu, drained and pressed

- 2 tablespoons soy sauce or tamari

- 1 tablespoon rice vinegar

- 1 tablespoon honey or maple syrup

- 1 tablespoon sesame oil

- 2 cloves garlic, minced

- 1 tablespoon fresh ginger, minced

- 1 tablespoon cornstarch

- 2 tablespoons olive oil

- 1 red bell pepper, thinly sliced

- 1 yellow bell pepper, thinly sliced

- 1 cup broccoli florets

- 1 cup snap peas

- 2 green onions, thinly sliced

- Cooked brown rice or quinoa for serving

Instructions:

1. Cut the pressed tofu into cubes and place them in a bowl. In a separate bowl, whisk together soy sauce or tamari, rice vinegar, honey or maple syrup, sesame oil, minced garlic, minced ginger, and cornstarch to make the sauce.

2. Pour the sauce over the tofu cubes and toss to coat. Let marinate for 10 minutes.

3. Heat olive oil in a large skillet or wok over medium-high heat. Add marinated tofu cubes and cook for 5-7 minutes until golden brown and crispy. Remove from skillet and set aside.

4. In the same skillet, add sliced bell peppers, broccoli florets, snap peas, and thinly sliced green onions. Stir-fry for 5-7 minutes until vegetables are tender-crisp.

5. Return cooked tofu to the skillet and toss everything together.

6. Serve hot over cooked brown rice or quinoa. Enjoy this flavourful and nutritious Asian-inspired tofu bowl!

Nutritional Information per Serving (without rice or quinoa):

- Calories: 280

- Protein: 15g

- Carbohydrates: 20g

- Fat: 15g

- Fiber: 5g

14. Mexican Quinoa Stuffed Bell Peppers

Prep Time: 20 minutes
Cooking Time: 30 minutes
Serving Size: 4

Ingredients:

- 1 cup quinoa, rinsed

- 2 cups water or vegetable broth

- 4 bell peppers (any colour), halved and seeds removed

- 1 can (15 oz) black beans, drained and rinsed

- 1 cup corn kernels (fresh, canned, or frozen)

- 1 cup cherry tomatoes, halved

- ½ cup red onion, diced

- ¼ cup fresh cilantro, chopped

- 1 teaspoon ground cumin

- 1 teaspoon chili powder

- Salt and pepper to taste

- 1 cup shredded cheese (cheddar, Monterey Jack, or a blend)

- Optional toppings: avocado slices, Greek yogurt, salsa

Instructions:

1. Preheat oven to 375°F (190°C). In a medium saucepan, bring the water or vegetable broth to a boil. Add the quinoa, reduce heat to low, cover, and simmer for 15 minutes or until all the liquid is absorbed.

2. In a large mixing bowl, combine the cooked quinoa, black beans, corn kernels, halved cherry tomatoes, diced red onion, chopped cilantro, ground cumin, chili powder, salt, and pepper.

3. Spoon the quinoa mixture evenly into each halved bell pepper, pressing down gently to pack the filling.

4. Place stuffed bell peppers in a baking dish and cover with aluminium foil. Bake in the preheated oven for 25 minutes.

5. Remove the foil and sprinkle shredded cheese over the top of each stuffed bell pepper. Return to the oven and bake for an additional 5 minutes or until the cheese is melted and bubbly.

6. Remove from the oven and let cool for a few minutes before serving.

7. Garnish with avocado slices, Greek yogurt, salsa, or your favourite toppings if desired.

8. Enjoy these flavourful and nutritious Mexican quinoa stuffed bell peppers as a satisfying lunch option!

Nutritional Information per Serving (1/4 of the recipe):

- Calories: 350

- Protein: 15g

- Carbohydrates: 45g

- Fat: 12g

- Fiber: 10g

15. Pesto Chicken and Vegetable Pasta

Prep Time: 20 minutes
Cooking Time: 20 minutes
Serving Size: 4

Ingredients:

- 8 oz whole wheat pasta (spaghetti, penne, or fusilli)

- 2 boneless, skinless chicken breasts, cut into cubes

- 2 tablespoons olive oil

- Salt and pepper to taste

- 1 cup cherry tomatoes, halved

- 1 cup broccoli florets

- ½ cup sliced mushrooms

- ¼ cup prepared pesto sauce

- Grated Parmesan cheese for serving

Instructions:

1. Cook the whole wheat pasta according to package instructions until al dente. Drain and set aside.

2. Heat olive oil in a large skillet over medium-high heat. Season the cubed chicken breasts with salt and pepper, then add them to the skillet. Cook for 5-7 minutes until golden brown and cooked through.

3. Add cherry tomatoes, broccoli florets, and sliced mushrooms to the skillet with the cooked chicken. Cook for an additional 5 minutes until vegetables are tender.

4. Stir in prepared pesto sauce and cooked pasta, tossing everything together until evenly coated.

5. Serve hot, garnished with grated Parmesan cheese if desired. Enjoy this delicious and satisfying pesto chicken and vegetable pasta for lunch!

Nutritional Information per Serving:

- Calories: 380

- Protein: 25g

- Carbohydrates: 40g

- Fat: 15g

- Fiber: 8g

16. Salmon and Asparagus Foil Packets

Prep Time: 15 minutes
Cooking Time: 20 minutes
Serving Size: 2

Ingredients:

- 2 salmon fillets (6 oz each)
- 1 bunch asparagus, trimmed
- 2 tablespoons olive oil
- 2 cloves garlic, minced
- 1 lemon, thinly sliced
- Salt and pepper to taste
- Fresh dill for garnish

Instructions:

1. Preheat oven to 375°F (190°C). Cut two large pieces of aluminium foil and place them on a flat surface.

2. Place one salmon fillet in the centre of each piece of foil. Arrange asparagus spears around the salmon.

3. Drizzle olive oil over the salmon and asparagus. Sprinkle minced garlic over the top, then season with salt and pepper to taste.

4. Place lemon slices on top of each salmon fillet.

5. Fold the sides of the foil over the salmon and asparagus, creating a sealed packet.

6. Place foil packets on a baking sheet and bake in the preheated oven for 18-20 minutes, or until salmon is cooked through and asparagus is tender.

7. Carefully open the foil packets and transfer the salmon and asparagus to serving plates.

8. Garnish with fresh dill before serving. Enjoy this easy and flavourful salmon and asparagus foil packet for lunch!

Nutritional Information per Serving:

- Calories: 350

- Protein: 30g

- Carbohydrates: 10g

- Fat: 20g

- Fiber: 5g

17. Veggie and Hummus Wrap

Prep Time: 10 minutes
Cooking Time: 0 minutes
Serving Size: 2

Ingredients:

- 4 large whole wheat tortillas

- ½ cup hummus (store-bought or homemade)

- 1 cup mixed salad greens

- 1 cucumber, sliced

- 1 bell pepper, thinly sliced

- 1 carrot, julienned

- ¼ cup red onion, thinly sliced

- Salt and pepper to taste

Instructions:

1. Lay out the tortillas on a clean surface. Spread a generous layer of hummus over each tortilla.

2. Divide the mixed salad greens, sliced cucumber, sliced bell pepper, julienned carrot, and thinly sliced red onion evenly among the tortillas.

3. Season with salt and pepper to taste.

4. Roll up each tortilla tightly, folding in the sides as you go to create a wrap.

5. Slice each wrap in half diagonally and serve immediately, or wrap in parchment paper for a portable lunch option.

Nutritional Information per Serving (1 wrap):

- Calories: 250

- Protein: 10g

- Carbohydrates: 35g

- Fat: 10g

- Fiber: 8g

18. Eggplant and Tomato Panini

Prep Time: 15 minutes
Cooking Time: 15 minutes
Serving Size: 2

Ingredients:

- 1 large eggplant, sliced into rounds

- 1 tomato, sliced

- 4 slices whole grain bread

- 4 slices mozzarella cheese

- ¼ cup fresh basil leaves

- 2 tablespoons olive oil

- Salt and pepper to taste

Instructions:

1. Preheat a panini press or grill pan over medium-high heat.

2. Brush eggplant slices with olive oil and season with salt and pepper.

3. Place eggplant slices on the panini press or grill pan and cook for 3-4 minutes on each side, until tender and grill marks appear.

4. Assemble the sandwiches by layering eggplant slices, tomato slices, mozzarella cheese, and fresh basil leaves between two slices of whole grain bread.

5. Brush the outsides of the sandwiches with olive oil.

6. Place sandwiches on the panini press or grill pan and cook for 5-6 minutes, until bread is golden brown and cheese is melted.

7. Remove sandwiches from the panini press or grill pan, slice in half, and serve hot. Enjoy this delicious and satisfying eggplant and tomato panini for lunch!

Nutritional Information per Serving (1 sandwich):

- Calories: 350

- Protein: 15g

- Carbohydrates: 35g

- Fat: 15g

- Fiber: 8g

19. Turkey and Vegetable Lettuce Wraps

Prep Time: 15 minutes
Cooking Time: 10 minutes
Serving Size: 2

Ingredients:

- 8 large lettuce leaves (such as romaine or butter lettuce)

- 8 oz lean ground turkey

- 1 tablespoon olive oil

- ½ cup bell pepper, diced

- ½ cup zucchini, diced

- ½ cup carrot, grated

- 2 cloves garlic, minced

- 2 tablespoons soy sauce or tamari

- 1 tablespoon hoisin sauce

- 1 teaspoon sesame oil

- 2 green onions, thinly sliced

- Optional toppings: chopped peanuts, cilantro, Sriracha

Instructions:

1. Heat olive oil in a large skillet over medium heat. Add minced garlic and cook for 1 minute until fragrant.

2. Add ground turkey to the skillet and cook until browned, breaking it up with a spoon, about 5-7 minutes.

3. Add diced bell pepper, diced zucchini, and grated carrot to the skillet. Cook for an additional 3-4 minutes until vegetables are tender.

4. Stir in soy sauce or tamari, hoisin sauce, and sesame oil. Cook for 1-2 minutes, stirring occasionally.

5. Remove skillet from heat and stir in thinly sliced green onions.

6. Spoon turkey and vegetable mixture onto lettuce leaves, dividing evenly among them.

7. Garnish with chopped peanuts, cilantro, and Sriracha if desired.

8. Roll up each lettuce leaf and secure with toothpicks if needed.

9. Serve immediately and enjoy these flavourful and satisfying turkey and vegetable lettuce wraps for lunch!

Nutritional Information per Serving (4 lettuce wraps):

- Calories: 280

- Protein: 20g

- Carbohydrates: 15g

- Fat: 15g

- Fiber: 5g

20. Veggie and Brown Rice Bowl

Prep Time: 20 minutes
Cooking Time: 40 minutes
Serving Size: 4

Ingredients:

- 2 cups cooked brown rice

- 1 can (15 oz) black beans, drained and rinsed

- 1 cup corn kernels (fresh, canned, or frozen)

- 1 red bell pepper, diced

- 1 avocado, diced

- ¼ cup red onion, finely chopped

- ¼ cup fresh cilantro, chopped

- Juice of 1 lime

- 2 tablespoons olive oil

- Salt and pepper to taste

Instructions:

1. In a large mixing bowl, combine the cooked brown rice, black beans, corn kernels, diced red bell Rpepper, diced avocado, chopped red onion, and chopped cilantro.

2. In a small bowl, whisk together the lime juice, olive oil, salt, and pepper to make the dressing.

3. Pour the dressing over the rice and vegetable mixture and toss gently to coat.

4. Divide the mixture among serving bowls and serve immediately.

5. Enjoy this delicious and nutritious veggie and brown rice bowl for lunch!

Nutritional Information per Serving:

- Calories: 320

- Protein: 12g

- Carbohydrates: 45g

- Fat: 12g

- Fiber: 10g

CHAPTER 5

DINER RECIPES

1. Grilled Lemon Herb Chicken

Prep Time: 10 minutes

Cook Time: 15 minutes

Serving Size: 4

Ingredients:

- 4 boneless, skinless chicken breasts
- 2 tablespoons olive oil
- 2 cloves garlic, minced
- 1 lemon, juiced and zested
- 2 teaspoons dried oregano
- 1 teaspoon dried thyme
- Salt and pepper to taste

Instructions:

1. In a small bowl, whisk together olive oil, garlic, lemon juice, lemon zest, oregano, thyme, salt, and pepper.

2. Place chicken breasts in a shallow dish and pour the marinade over them, ensuring they are evenly coated. Cover and refrigerate for at least 30 minutes.

3. Preheat grill to medium-high heat. Remove chicken from marinade and discard excess marinade.

4. Grill chicken breasts for 6-7 minutes per side, or until cooked through and no longer pink in the centre.

5. Serve hot with your choice of vegetables or salad.

Nutritional Information (per serving):

- Calories: 250

- Protein: 30g

- Carbohydrates: 2g

- Fat: 14g

2. Baked Salmon with Roasted Vegetables

Prep Time: 15 minutes

Cook Time: 20 minutes

Serving Size: 4

Ingredients:

- 4 salmon fillets

- 2 tablespoons olive oil

- 2 cloves garlic, minced

- 1 teaspoon dried dill

- 1 teaspoon paprika

- Salt and pepper to taste

- 2 cups assorted vegetables (bell peppers, zucchini, cherry tomatoes, etc.)

Instructions:

1. Preheat oven to 400°F (200°C). Line a baking sheet with parchment paper.

2. In a small bowl, mix together olive oil, garlic, dill, paprika, salt, and pepper.

3. Place salmon fillets on the prepared baking sheet. Brush with the olive oil mixture, coating both sides.

4. Arrange assorted vegetables around the salmon on the baking sheet.

5. Bake in the preheated oven for 15-20 minutes, or until salmon is cooked through and vegetables are tender.

6. Serve hot, garnished with fresh herbs if desired.

Nutritional Information (per serving):

- Calories: 300

- Protein: 25g

- Carbohydrates: 8g

- Fat: 18g

3. Quinoa Stuffed Bell Peppers

Prep Time: 20 minutes

Cook Time: 30 minutes

Serving Size: 4

Ingredients:

- 4 large bell peppers, halved and seeds removed
- 1 cup quinoa, rinsed
- 2 cups vegetable broth
- 1 onion, diced
- 2 cloves garlic, minced
- 1 can (15 oz) black beans, drained and rinsed
- 1 can (15 oz) diced tomatoes, drained
- 1 teaspoon cumin
- 1 teaspoon chili powder
- Salt and pepper to taste
- 1 cup shredded cheese (optional)

Instructions:

1. Preheat oven to 375°F (190°C). Place bell pepper halves cut side up in a baking dish.

2. In a medium saucepan, bring vegetable broth to a boil. Add quinoa, reduce heat to low, cover, and simmer for 15-20 minutes, or until quinoa is cooked and liquid is absorbed.

3. In a skillet, heat olive oil over medium heat. Add onion and garlic, and sauté until softened.

4. Stir in black beans, diced tomatoes, cumin, chili powder, salt, and pepper. Cook for 5 minutes.

5. Remove skillet from heat and stir in cooked quinoa.

6. Spoon quinoa mixture into bell pepper halves, pressing down gently to pack the filling.

7. If using cheese, sprinkle it over the stuffed peppers.

8. Cover baking dish with foil and bake for 25-30 minutes, or until peppers are tender.

9. Serve hot, garnished with fresh herbs if desired.

Nutritional Information (per serving without cheese):

- Calories: 320

- Protein: 12g

- Carbohydrates: 55g

- Fat: 6g

4. Turkey and Vegetable Stir-Fry

Prep Time: 15 minutes

Cook Time: 15 minutes

Serving Size: 4

Ingredients:

- 1 lb lean ground turkey

- 2 tablespoons soy sauce (or tamari for gluten-free option)

- 1 tablespoon sesame oil

- 2 cloves garlic, minced

- 1 teaspoon ginger, minced

- 1 onion, sliced

- 2 cups mixed vegetables (bell peppers, broccoli, carrots, snap peas, etc.)

- 2 green onions, sliced

- Cooked brown rice or cauliflower rice, for serving

Instructions:

1. In a small bowl, mix together soy sauce and sesame oil. Set aside.

2. In a large skillet or wok, heat olive oil over medium heat. Add ground turkey and cook until browned, breaking it apart with a spoon.

3. Add garlic and ginger to the skillet, and cook for 1 minute until fragrant.

4. Add sliced onion and mixed vegetables to the skillet. Stir-fry for 5-7 minutes, or until vegetables are tender-crisp.

5. Pour the soy sauce mixture over the turkey and vegetables. Stir well to combine and coat everything evenly.

6. Cook for an additional 2-3 minutes, allowing the flavours to meld together.

7. Remove from heat and garnish with sliced green onions.

8. Serve hot over cooked brown rice or cauliflower rice.

Nutritional Information (per serving):

- Calories: 280
- Protein: 24g
- Carbohydrates: 12g
- Fat: 14g

5. Eggplant Parmesan

Prep Time: 30 minutes

Cook Time: 45 minutes

Serving Size: 4

Ingredients:

- 2 medium eggplants, sliced into ½-inch rounds
- 2 eggs, beaten
- 1 cup whole wheat breadcrumbs
- 1 cup grated Parmesan cheese
- 2 cups marinara sauce
- 1 cup shredded mozzarella cheese
- Fresh basil leaves, for garnish
- Olive oil for frying
- Salt and pepper to taste

Instructions:

1. Preheat oven to 375°F (190°C). Grease a baking sheet with olive oil.

2. Season eggplant slices with salt and pepper. Dip each slice into beaten eggs, then coat with breadcrumbs mixed with grated Parmesan cheese.

3. Place breaded eggplant slices on the prepared baking sheet. Bake for 15-20 minutes, or until golden brown and crispy.

4. Spread a thin layer of marinara sauce in the bottom of a baking dish.

5. Arrange half of the baked eggplant slices in the baking dish, overlapping slightly.

6. Top with half of the remaining marinara sauce and half of the shredded mozzarella cheese.

7. Repeat the layers with the remaining eggplant slices, marinara sauce, and mozzarella cheese.

8. Bake for 25-30 minutes, or until cheese is melted and bubbly.

9. Garnish with fresh basil leaves before serving.

Nutritional Information (per serving):

- Calories: 320
- Protein: 18g
- Carbohydrates: 25g
- Fat: 16g

6. Lentil and Vegetable Curry

Prep Time: 15 minutes

Cook Time: 30 minutes

Serving Size: 4

Ingredients:

- 1 cup dried lentils, rinsed
- 4 cups vegetable broth
- 1 onion, diced
- 2 cloves garlic, minced
- 1 tablespoon curry powder
- 1 teaspoon ground turmeric
- 1 teaspoon ground cumin
- 1 teaspoon ground coriander
- 1 can (15 oz) diced tomatoes, undrained
- 2 cups mixed vegetables (bell peppers, carrots, cauliflower, etc.)
- 1 can (15 oz) coconut milk
- Salt and pepper to taste
- Fresh cilantro, for garnish

- Cooked brown rice or quinoa, for serving

Instructions:

1. In a large pot, combine lentils and vegetable broth. Bring to a boil, then reduce heat to low and simmer for 15-20 minutes, or until lentils are tender.

2. In a skillet, heat olive oil over medium heat. Add onion and garlic, and sauté until softened.

3. Stir in curry powder, turmeric, cumin, and coriander. Cook for 1 minute until fragrant.

4. Add diced tomatoes (with their juices) and mixed vegetables to the skillet. Cook for 5 minutes.

5. Add cooked lentils and coconut milk to the skillet. Stir well to combine.

6. Simmer the curry for 10-15 minutes, or until vegetables are tender and flavours are well combined.

7. Season with salt and pepper to taste.

8. Serve hot over cooked brown rice or quinoa, garnished with fresh cilantro.

Nutritional Information (per serving without rice/quinoa):

- Calories: 320

- Protein: 15g

- Carbohydrates: 30g

- Fat: 18g

7. Turkey Meatball and Vegetable Skewers

Prep Time: 20 minutes

Cook Time: 15 minutes

Serving Size: 4

Ingredients:

- 1 lb lean ground turkey
- 1 egg
- ½ cup breadcrumbs
- 2 cloves garlic, minced
- 1 teaspoon dried oregano
- 1 teaspoon dried basil
- Salt and pepper to taste
- 2 bell peppers, cut into chunks
- 1 zucchini, sliced
- 1 onion, cut into wedges
- Wooden or metal skewers

Instructions:

1. Preheat grill or grill pan to medium-high heat.
2. In a large bowl, combine ground turkey, egg, breadcrumbs, garlic, oregano, basil, salt, and pepper. Mix until well combined.
3. Shape turkey mixture into small meatballs.

4. Thread turkey meatballs onto skewers, alternating with chunks of bell peppers, zucchini slices, and onion wedges.

5. Lightly brush skewers with olive oil.

6. Grill skewers for 12-15 minutes, turning occasionally, until turkey meatballs are cooked through and vegetables are tender.

7. Serve hot with your favourite dipping sauce or tzatziki.

Nutritional Information (per serving):

- Calories: 250

- Protein: 22g

- Carbohydrates: 15g

- Fat: 10g

8. Cauliflower Fried Rice

Prep Time: 15 minutes

Cook Time: 15 minutes

Serving Size: 4

Ingredients:

- 1 head cauliflower, grated or finely chopped

- 2 tablespoons sesame oil

- 2 cloves garlic, minced

- 1 onion, diced

- 2 carrots, diced

- 1 cup frozen peas

- 2 eggs, beaten

- 3 tablespoons soy sauce (or tamari for gluten-free option)

- 2 green onions, sliced

- Salt and pepper to taste

Instructions:

1. In a large skillet or wok, heat sesame oil over medium heat.

2. Add minced garlic and diced onion to the skillet. Sauté until softened.

3. Add diced carrots and frozen peas to the skillet. Cook for 3-4 minutes, or until vegetables are tender.

4. Push the vegetables to one side of the skillet. Pour beaten eggs into the empty side of the skillet. Scramble the eggs until cooked through, then mix with the vegetables.

5. Add grated cauliflower to the skillet. Stir well to combine with the vegetables and eggs.

6. Pour soy sauce over the cauliflower mixture. Season with salt and pepper to taste. Stir-fry for an additional 3-4 minutes.

7. Garnish with sliced green onions before serving.

Nutritional Information (per serving):

- Calories: 180

- Protein: 8g

- Carbohydrates: 15g

- Fat: 10g

9. Lemon Garlic Shrimp with Zucchini Noodles

Prep Time: 15 minutes

Cook Time: 10 minutes

Serving Size: 4

Ingredients:

- 1 lb large shrimp, peeled and deveined

- 2 tablespoons olive oil

- 4 cloves garlic, minced

- 1 lemon, juiced and zested

- 4 medium zucchinis, spiralized into noodles

- Salt and pepper to taste

- Fresh parsley, for garnish

Instructions:

1. In a large skillet, heat olive oil over medium heat. Add minced garlic and cook until fragrant, about 1 minute.

2. Add shrimp to the skillet in a single layer. Cook for 2-3 minutes per side, or until pink and opaque.

3. Stir in lemon juice and lemon zest, coating the shrimp evenly.

4. Add spiralized zucchini noodles to the skillet. Toss with the shrimp and garlic mixture until heated through, about 2-3 minutes.

5. Season with salt and pepper to taste.

6. Garnish with fresh parsley before serving.

Nutritional Information (per serving):

- Calories: 180

- Protein: 25g

- Carbohydrates: 8g

- Fat: 8g

10. Spaghetti Squash with Turkey Bolognese

Prep Time: 20 minutes

Cook Time: 1 hour

Serving Size: 4

Ingredients:

- 1 large spaghetti squash

- 1 lb lean ground turkey

- 1 onion, diced

- 2 cloves garlic, minced

- 1 can (15 oz) crushed tomatoes

- 1 teaspoon dried oregano

- 1 teaspoon dried basil

- Salt and pepper to taste

- Fresh parsley, for garnish

- Grated Parmesan cheese (optional)

Instructions:

1. Preheat oven to 375°F (190°C). Cut spaghetti squash in half lengthwise and remove seeds with a spoon.

2. Place squash halves cut side down on a baking sheet lined with parchment paper. Bake for 45-60 minutes, or until squash is tender and easily pierced with a fork.

3. While squash is baking, heat olive oil in a large skillet over medium heat. Add ground turkey, onion, and garlic. Cook until turkey is browned and onions are softened.

4. Stir in crushed tomatoes, oregano, basil, salt, and pepper. Simmer for 15-20 minutes, allowing flavours to meld together.

5. Once spaghetti squash is cooked, use a fork to scrape the flesh into strands.

6. Serve spaghetti squash topped with turkey Bolognese sauce.

7. Garnish with fresh parsley and grated Parmesan cheese, if desired.

Nutritional Information (per serving without cheese):

- Calories: 280

- Protein: 24g

- Carbohydrates: 20g

- Fat: 12g

11. Veggie Stir-Fry with Tofu

Prep Time: 20 minutes

Cook Time: 15 minutes

Serving Size: 4

Ingredients:

- 1 block (14 oz) firm tofu, pressed and cubed

- 2 tablespoons soy sauce (or tamari for gluten-free option)

- 1 tablespoon sesame oil

- 2 cloves garlic, minced

- 1 teaspoon ginger, minced

- 1 onion, sliced

- 2 cups mixed vegetables (bell peppers, broccoli, snap peas, carrots, etc.)

- 2 green onions, sliced

- Cooked brown rice or quinoa, for serving

Instructions:

1. In a small bowl, combine cubed tofu with soy sauce. Set aside to marinate for 10-15 minutes.

2. Heat sesame oil in a large skillet or wok over medium heat.

3. Add minced garlic and ginger to the skillet. Sauté until fragrant, about 1 minute.

4. Add sliced onion to the skillet. Cook until softened.

5. Add marinated tofu to the skillet, reserving any excess marinade. Cook until tofu is lightly browned on all sides.

6. Add mixed vegetables to the skillet. Stir-fry until vegetables are tender-crisp.

7. Pour reserved marinade over the tofu and vegetables. Stir well to combine.

8. Cook for an additional 2-3 minutes, allowing flavours to meld together.

9. Serve hot over cooked brown rice or quinoa, garnished with sliced green onions.

Nutritional Information (per serving without rice/quinoa):

- Calories: 220

- Protein: 18g

- Carbohydrates: 15g

- Fat: 10g

12. Lemon Garlic Roasted Chicken with Asparagus

Prep Time: 15 minutes

Cook Time: 25 minutes

Serving Size: 4

Ingredients:

- 4 boneless, skinless chicken breasts
- 2 tablespoons olive oil
- 4 cloves garlic, minced
- 1 lemon, juiced and zested
- 1 teaspoon dried thyme
- 1 teaspoon dried rosemary
- Salt and pepper to taste
- 1 bunch asparagus, trimmed
- Fresh parsley, for garnish

Instructions:

1. Preheat oven to 400°F (200°C). Line a baking sheet with parchment paper.

2. In a small bowl, whisk together olive oil, garlic, lemon juice, lemon zest, thyme, rosemary, salt, and pepper.

3. Place chicken breasts on the prepared baking sheet. Brush with the olive oil mixture, coating both sides.

4. Arrange trimmed asparagus around the chicken on the baking sheet.

5. Roast in the preheated oven for 20-25 minutes, or until chicken is cooked through and asparagus is tender.

6. Serve hot, garnished with fresh parsley.

Nutritional Information (per serving):

- Calories: 280

- Protein: 30g

- Carbohydrates: 6g

- Fat: 14g

13. Moroccan Spiced Chickpea Stew

Prep Time: 15 minutes

Cook Time: 30 minutes

Serving Size: 4

Ingredients:

- 2 tablespoons olive oil

- 1 onion, diced

- 2 cloves garlic, minced

- 1 teaspoon ground cumin

- 1 teaspoon ground coriander

- ½ teaspoon ground cinnamon

- ½ teaspoon ground turmeric

- 1 can (15 oz) chickpeas, drained and rinsed

- 1 can (15 oz) diced tomatoes, undrained

- 2 cups vegetable broth

- 2 cups spinach leaves

- Salt and pepper to taste

- Fresh cilantro, for garnish

- Cooked couscous or quinoa, for serving

Instructions:

1. In a large pot, heat olive oil over medium heat. Add diced onion and minced garlic. Sauté until softened.

2. Stir in ground cumin, ground coriander, ground cinnamon, and ground turmeric. Cook for 1 minute until fragrant.

3. Add chickpeas, diced tomatoes, and vegetable broth to the pot. Bring to a simmer.

4. Simmer for 20-25 minutes, allowing flavours to meld together and stew to thicken.

5. Stir in spinach leaves and cook until wilted.

6. Season with salt and pepper to taste.

7. Serve hot over cooked couscous or quinoa, garnished with fresh cilantro.

Nutritional Information (per serving without couscous/quinoa):

- Calories: 250

- Protein: 10g

- Carbohydrates: 30g

- Fat: 10g

14. Teriyaki Tofu and Vegetable Stir-Fry

Prep Time: 20 minutes

Cook Time: 15 minutes

Serving Size: 4

Ingredients:

- 1 block (14 oz) firm tofu, pressed and cubed

- ½ cup teriyaki sauce

- 2 tablespoons olive oil

- 2 cloves garlic, minced

- 1 onion, sliced

- 2 bell peppers, sliced

- 1 cup broccoli florets

- 1 cup snap peas

- Cooked brown rice or quinoa, for serving

- Sesame seeds, for garnish

Instructions:

1. In a shallow dish, marinate cubed tofu in teriyaki sauce for 10-15 minutes.

2. In a large skillet or wok, heat olive oil over medium heat. Add minced garlic and cook until fragrant.

3. Add sliced onion, bell peppers, broccoli florets, and snap peas to the skillet. Stir-fry until vegetables are tender-crisp.

4. Push vegetables to one side of the skillet. Add marinated tofu to the empty side of the skillet. Cook until tofu is browned on all sides.

5. Combine tofu with vegetables in the skillet. Stir well to combine.

6. Serve hot over cooked brown rice or quinoa.

7. Garnish with sesame seeds before serving.

Nutritional Information (per serving without rice/quinoa):

- Calories: 220

- Protein: 15g

- Carbohydrates: 20g

- Fat: 10g

15. Mediterranean Baked Cod

Prep Time: 15 minutes

Cook Time: 20 minutes

Serving Size: 4

Ingredients:

- 4 cod fillets

- 2 tablespoons olive oil

- 2 cloves garlic, minced

- 1 lemon, juiced and zested
- 1 teaspoon dried oregano
- ½ teaspoon dried basil
- ½ teaspoon dried thyme
- Salt and pepper to taste
- ½ cup cherry tomatoes, halved
- ¼ cup Kalamata olives, pitted and sliced
- Fresh parsley, for garnish

Instructions:

1. Preheat oven to 400°F (200°C). Line a baking sheet with parchment paper.

2. In a small bowl, whisk together olive oil, garlic, lemon juice, lemon zest, oregano, basil, thyme, salt, and pepper.

3. Place cod fillets on the prepared baking sheet. Brush with the olive oil mixture, coating both sides.

4. Arrange cherry tomatoes and Kalamata olives around the cod fillets.

5. Bake in the preheated oven for 15-20 minutes, or until cod is cooked through and flakes easily with a fork.

6. Serve hot, garnished with fresh parsley.

Nutritional Information (per serving):

- Calories: 220
- Protein: 25g
- Carbohydrates: 5g
- Fat: 10g

16. Butternut Squash and Black Bean Enchiladas

Prep Time: 30 minutes

Cook Time: 30 minutes

Serving Size: 4

Ingredients:

- 1 butternut squash, peeled and diced
- 1 tablespoon olive oil
- 1 onion, diced
- 2 cloves garlic, minced
- 1 can (15 oz) black beans, drained and rinsed
- 1 cup corn kernels (fresh or frozen)
- 1 teaspoon ground cumin
- 1 teaspoon chili powder
- ½ teaspoon smoked paprika
- Salt and pepper to taste
- 8 whole wheat tortillas
- 1 cup enchilada sauce

- 1 cup shredded cheese (cheddar or Mexican blend)

- Fresh cilantro, for garnish

Instructions:

1. Preheat oven to 375°F (190°C). Grease a 9x13-inch baking dish with olive oil.

2. Place diced butternut squash on a baking sheet. Drizzle with olive oil and season with salt and pepper. Roast in the preheated oven for 20-25 minutes, or until squash is tender.

3. In a skillet, heat olive oil over medium heat. Add diced onion and minced garlic. Sauté until softened.

4. Stir in black beans, corn kernels, ground cumin, chili powder, smoked paprika, salt, and pepper. Cook for 5 minutes.

5. Add roasted butternut squash to the skillet. Stir well to combine.

6. Spoon the filling onto each whole wheat tortilla. Roll up and place seam side down in the prepared baking dish.

7. Pour enchilada sauce over the rolled tortillas. Sprinkle shredded cheese on top.

8. Bake in the preheated oven for 25-30 minutes, or until cheese is melted and bubbly.

9. Garnish with fresh cilantro before serving.

Nutritional Information (per serving without cheese):

- Calories: 300
- Protein: 10g
- Carbohydrates: 50g
- Fat: 8g

17. Greek Salad with Grilled Chicken

Prep Time: 20 minutes

Cook Time: 15 minutes

Serving Size: 4

Ingredients:

- 2 boneless, skinless chicken breasts
- 2 tablespoons olive oil
- 2 cloves garlic, minced
- 1 lemon, juiced and zested
- 1 teaspoon dried oregano
- Salt and pepper to taste
- 4 cups mixed greens (lettuce, spinach, arugula, etc.)
- 1 cucumber, sliced
- 1 bell pepper, sliced
- 1 cup cherry tomatoes, halved
- ½ cup Kalamata olives, pitted
- ½ cup feta cheese, crumbled

- Greek salad dressing (homemade or store-bought)

Instructions:

1. In a small bowl, whisk together olive oil, garlic, lemon juice, lemon zest, oregano, salt, and pepper.

2. Place chicken breasts in a shallow dish and pour the marinade over them, ensuring they are evenly coated. Cover and refrigerate for at least 30 minutes.

3. Preheat grill to medium-high heat. Remove chicken from marinade and discard excess marinade.

4. Grill chicken breasts for 6-7 minutes per side, or until cooked through and no longer pink in the centre.

5. Let chicken rest for a few minutes, then slice into strips.

6. In a large bowl, combine mixed greens, cucumber slices, bell pepper slices, cherry tomatoes, Kalamata olives, and feta cheese.

7. Arrange grilled chicken strips on top of the salad.

8. Drizzle Greek salad dressing over the salad and toss gently to coat.

9. Serve immediately.

Nutritional Information (per serving without dressing):

- Calories: 280

- Protein: 25g

- Carbohydrates: 10g

- Fat: 15g

18. Beef and Broccoli Stir-Fry

Prep Time: 20 minutes

Cook Time: 15 minutes

Serving Size: 4

Ingredients:

- 1 lb flank steak, thinly sliced against the grain
- ⅓ cup soy sauce (or tamari for gluten-free option)
- 2 tablespoons cornstarch
- 2 tablespoons brown sugar
- 2 tablespoons olive oil
- 2 cloves garlic, minced
- 1 teaspoon ginger, minced
- 2 cups broccoli florets
- Cooked brown rice or quinoa, for serving

Instructions:

1. In a small bowl, whisk together soy sauce, cornstarch, and brown sugar. Set aside.

2. Heat olive oil in a large skillet or wok over medium heat. Add minced garlic and ginger. Cook until fragrant.

3. Add sliced flank steak to the skillet. Stir-fry until browned and cooked to desired doneness.

4. Add broccoli florets to the skillet. Stir-fry until tender-crisp.

5. Pour the soy sauce mixture over the beef and broccoli in the skillet. Stir well to coat everything evenly.

6. Cook for an additional 2-3 minutes, allowing the sauce to thicken.

7. Serve hot over cooked brown rice or quinoa.

Nutritional Information (per serving without rice/quinoa):

- Calories: 320

- Protein: 25g

- Carbohydrates: 10g

- Fat: 15g

19. Spinach and Mushroom Stuffed Chicken Breast

Prep Time: 20 minutes

Cook Time: 25 minutes

Serving Size: 4

Ingredients:

- 4 boneless, skinless chicken breasts

- 1 tablespoon olive oil

- 2 cloves garlic, minced

- 2 cups baby spinach leaves

- 1 cup mushrooms, sliced

- ½ cup shredded mozzarella cheese

- Salt and pepper to taste

- Toothpicks

Instructions:

1. Preheat oven to 375°F (190°C). Grease a baking dish with olive oil.

2. In a skillet, heat olive oil over medium heat. Add minced garlic and cook until fragrant.

3. Add baby spinach leaves to the skillet. Cook until wilted.

4. Add sliced mushrooms to the skillet. Cook until softened.

5. Season chicken breasts with salt and pepper. Use a sharp knife to cut a pocket into the side of each chicken breast.

6. Stuff each chicken breast with the spinach and mushroom mixture, then sprinkle shredded mozzarella cheese on top.

7. Use toothpicks to secure the openings of the chicken breasts.

8. Place stuffed chicken breasts in the prepared baking dish.

9. Bake in the preheated oven for 20-25 minutes, or until chicken is cooked through and cheese is melted.

10. Remove toothpicks before serving.

Nutritional Information (per serving):

- Calories: 280

- Protein: 30g

- Carbohydrates: 4g

- Fat: 14g

20. Vegetable and Lentil Soup

Prep Time: 15 minutes

Cook Time: 30 minutes

Serving Size: 4

Ingredients:

- 1 tablespoon olive oil

- 1 onion, diced

- 2 cloves garlic, minced

- 2 carrots, diced

- 2 celery stalks, diced

- 1 cup dried green lentils, rinsed

- 4 cups vegetable broth

- 1 can (15 oz) diced tomatoes, undrained

- 2 cups spinach leaves

- 1 teaspoon dried thyme

- Salt and pepper to taste

- Fresh parsley, for garnish

Instructions:

1. In a large pot, heat olive oil over medium heat. Add diced onion and minced garlic. Sauté until softened.

2. Add diced carrots and celery to the pot. Cook for 5 minutes.

3. Stir in dried green lentils, vegetable broth, diced tomatoes, dried thyme, salt, and pepper.

4. Bring soup to a boil, then reduce heat to low and simmer for 20-25 minutes, or until lentils are tender.

5. Stir in spinach leaves and cook until wilted.

6. Season with additional salt and pepper to taste.

7. Serve hot, garnished with fresh parsley.

Nutritional Information (per serving):

- Calories: 250

- Protein: 15g

- Carbohydrates: 40g

- Fat: 5g

CHAPTER 6

SNACKS RECIPES

1. Avocado and Tomato Toast

Prep Time: 5 minutes
Cooking Time: 5 minutes
Serving Size: 1 toast

Ingredients:

- 1 slice of whole grain bread

- ½ ripe avocado

- 1 small tomato, sliced

- Salt and pepper to taste

- Optional toppings: red pepper flakes, chopped cilantro

Instructions:

1. Toast the whole grain bread until golden brown.

2. Mash the ripe avocado in a bowl and season with salt and pepper.

3. Spread the mashed avocado evenly onto the toasted bread.

4. Top with sliced tomatoes and any optional toppings of your choice.

5. Serve immediately and enjoy!

Nutritional Information (per serving):

- Calories: 200
- Protein: 5g
- Carbohydrates: 20g
- Fat: 12g
- Fiber: 6g

2. Greek Yogurt with Berries

Prep Time: 5 minutes
Serving Size: 1 bowl

Ingredients:

- ½ cup Greek yogurt
- ½ cup mixed berries (strawberries, blueberries, raspberries)
- 1 tablespoon honey or maple syrup (optional)
- 1 tablespoon chopped nuts (almonds, walnuts, or pistachios)

Instructions:

1. In a bowl, spoon the Greek yogurt.
2. Wash the berries and place them on top of the yogurt.
3. Drizzle with honey or maple syrup if desired.
4. Sprinkle chopped nuts over the yogurt and berries.
5. Serve chilled and enjoy!

Nutritional Information (per serving):

- Calories: 180

- Protein: 15g

- Carbohydrates: 20g

- Fat: 6g

- Fiber: 5g

3. Veggie Sticks with Hummus

Prep Time: 10 minutes
Serving Size: 1 serving

Ingredients:

- 1 medium carrot, cut into sticks

- 1 medium cucumber, cut into sticks

- 2 tablespoons hummus

Instructions:

1. Wash and cut the carrot and cucumber into sticks.

2. Place the veggie sticks on a plate.

3. Serve with hummus for dipping.

4. Enjoy the crunchy and flavourful snack!

Nutritional Information (per serving):

- Calories: 100

- Protein: 3g

- Carbohydrates: 15g

- Fat: 5g

- Fiber: 6g

4. Apple Slices with Almond Butter

Prep Time: 5 minutes
Serving Size: 1 apple

Ingredients:

- 1 apple, sliced

- 2 tablespoons almond butter

- Cinnamon (optional)

Instructions:

1. Wash and slice the apple into thin wedges.

2. Spread almond butter on each apple slice.

3. Sprinkle with cinnamon if desired.

4. Arrange on a plate and serve immediately.

Nutritional Information (per serving):

- Calories: 180

- Protein: 4g

- Carbohydrates: 25g

- Fat: 9g

- Fiber: 6g

5. Cottage Cheese with Pineapple

Prep Time: 5 minutes
Serving Size: 1/2 cup

Ingredients:

- ½ cup cottage cheese

- ½ cup fresh pineapple chunks

Instructions:

1. Spoon cottage cheese into a bowl.

2. Add fresh pineapple chunks on top.

3. Mix gently and enjoy the creamy and sweet combination.

Nutritional Information (per serving):

- Calories: 120

- Protein: 14g

- Carbohydrates: 15g

- Fat: 2g

- Fiber: 2g

6. Rice Cake with Almond Butter and Banana

Prep Time: 5 minutes
Serving Size: 1 rice cake

Ingredients:

- 1 rice cake

- 1 tablespoon almond butter

- ½ banana, sliced
- Honey (optional)

Instructions:

1. Spread almond butter evenly on the rice cake.
2. Top with banana slices.
3. Drizzle with honey if desired.
4. Serve immediately and enjoy the crunchy and creamy snack.

Nutritional Information (per serving):

- Calories: 140
- Protein: 3g
- Carbohydrates: 20g
- Fat: 6g
- Fiber: 3g

7. Hard-Boiled Eggs with Cherry Tomatoes

Prep Time: 10 minutes
Cooking Time: 10 minutes
Serving Size: 2 eggs

Ingredients:

- 2 large eggs
- ½ cup cherry tomatoes
- Salt and pepper to taste

Instructions:

1. Place the eggs in a saucepan and cover with water.

2. Bring the water to a boil, then reduce the heat and simmer for 8-10 minutes.

3. Once cooked, transfer the eggs to a bowl of ice water to cool.

4. Peel the eggs and slice them in half.

5. Serve with cherry tomatoes on the side.

6. Season with salt and pepper to taste.

7. Enjoy this protein-packed snack!

Nutritional Information (per serving):

- Calories: 140

- Protein: 12g

- Carbohydrates: 3g

- Fat: 9g

- Fiber: 1g

8. Edamame with Sea Salt

Prep Time: 5 minutes
Cooking Time: 5 minutes
Serving Size: ½ cup

Ingredients:

- 1 cup edamame (frozen or fresh)

- Sea salt to taste

Instructions:

1. If using frozen edamame, steam or boil them according to package instructions.

2. If using fresh edamame, boil them in salted water for 5 minutes, then drain.

3. Sprinkle the cooked edamame with sea salt.

4. Serve warm or chilled and enjoy as a nutritious snack.

Nutritional Information (per serving):

- Calories: 120

- Protein: 11g

- Carbohydrates: 8g

- Fat: 5g

- Fiber: 5g

9. Kale Chips

Prep Time: 10 minutes
Cooking Time: 20 minutes
Serving Size: 1 cup

Ingredients:

- 1 bunch kale, stems removed and leaves torn into bite-sized pieces

- 1 tablespoon olive oil

- Salt and pepper to taste

- Optional: nutritional yeast, garlic powder, paprika

Instructions:

1. Preheat the oven to 350°F (175°C).

2. In a large bowl, toss the kale leaves with olive oil until evenly coated.

3. Season with salt, pepper, and any optional seasonings of your choice.

4. Spread the kale in a single layer on a baking sheet lined with parchment paper.

5. Bake for 15-20 minutes, or until the kale is crispy and slightly browned.

6. Remove from the oven and let cool before serving.

7. Enjoy the crunchy and flavourful kale chips as a satisfying snack.

Nutritional Information (per serving):

- Calories: 50
- Protein: 2g
- Carbohydrates: 5g
- Fat: 3g
- Fiber: 2g

10. Quinoa Salad Cups

Prep Time: 15 minutes
Cooking Time: 15 minutes
Serving Size: 2 cups

Ingredients:

- 1 cup cooked quinoa

- ½ cup diced cucumber

- ½ cup diced bell pepper (red, yellow, or green)

- ¼ cup chopped fresh parsley

- 2 tablespoons lemon juice

- 1 tablespoon olive oil

- Salt and pepper to taste

- Optional: crumbled feta cheese, sliced olives, cherry tomatoes

Instructions:

1. In a large bowl, combine the cooked quinoa, diced cucumber, diced bell pepper, and chopped parsley.

2. Drizzle with lemon juice and olive oil, then season with salt and pepper.

3. Toss until all ingredients are well combined.

4. Spoon the quinoa salad into small cups or bowls for easy serving.

5. Garnish with optional toppings such as crumbled feta cheese, sliced olives, or cherry tomatoes.

6. Serve chilled or at room temperature and enjoy this refreshing and nutritious snack.

Nutritional Information (per serving):

- Calories: 180

- Protein: 5g

- Carbohydrates: 25g

- Fat: 7g

- Fiber: 4g

CHAPTER 7

DESSERT RECIPES

1. Berry Chia Seed Pudding

Prep Time: 5 minutes
Cooking Time: 0 minutes
Serving Size: 2

Ingredients:

- 1 cup unsweetened almond milk

- ¼ cup chia seeds

- ½ teaspoon vanilla extract

- 1 cup mixed berries (strawberries, blueberries, raspberries)

- Optional: Stevia or monk fruit sweetener to taste

Instructions:

1. In a bowl, whisk together almond milk, chia seeds, and vanilla extract.

2. Let the mixture sit for 5 minutes, then whisk again to prevent clumping.

3. Cover the bowl and refrigerate for at least 2 hours or overnight.

4. Before serving, stir the chia pudding to loosen it up.

5. Layer the chia pudding with mixed berries in serving glasses or bowls.

6. Optionally, sweeten with stevia or monk fruit sweetener to taste.

7. Serve chilled.

Nutritional Information (per serving):

- Calories: 150

- Total Fat: 8g

- Saturated Fat: 1g

- Carbohydrates: 15g

- Fiber: 10g

- Sugars: 3g

- Protein: 5g

2. Baked Apples with Cinnamon

Prep Time: 10 minutes
Cooking Time: 30 minutes
Serving Size: 2

Ingredients:

- 2 medium apples (such as Granny Smith or Honeycrisp)

- 1 tablespoon lemon juice

- 1 teaspoon ground cinnamon

- ¼ teaspoon ground nutmeg

- Optional: Stevia or monk fruit sweetener to taste

Instructions:

1. Preheat the oven to 375°F (190°C).

2. Core the apples and slice them into thin rings or chunks.

3. Toss the apple slices with lemon juice, cinnamon, and nutmeg until evenly coated.

4. Arrange the seasoned apple slices in a baking dish.

5. Optionally, sprinkle with stevia or monk fruit sweetener for added sweetness.

6. Bake in the preheated oven for 25-30 minutes or until the apples are tender.

7. Serve warm as is or with a dollop of Greek yogurt on top.

Nutritional Information (per serving):

- Calories: 80
- Total Fat: 0g
- Saturated Fat: 0g
- Carbohydrates: 22g
- Fiber: 5g
- Sugars: 16g
- Protein: 0g

3. Chocolate Avocado Mousse

Prep Time: 10 minutes
Cooking Time: 0 minutes
Serving Size: 2

Ingredients:

- 1 ripe avocado

- 2 tablespoons unsweetened cocoa powder

- 2 tablespoons honey or maple syrup

- ½ teaspoon vanilla extract

- Pinch of salt

- Optional toppings: Fresh berries, sliced almonds

Instructions:

1. Scoop the flesh of the avocado into a blender or food processor.

2. Add cocoa powder, honey or maple syrup, vanilla extract, and a pinch of salt.

3. Blend until smooth and creamy, scraping down the sides as needed.

4. Taste and adjust sweetness if necessary by adding more honey or maple syrup.

5. Transfer the mousse into serving bowls or glasses.

6. Refrigerate for at least 30 minutes to chill and set.

7. Serve topped with fresh berries and sliced almonds if desired.

Nutritional Information (per serving):

- Calories: 200
- Total Fat: 12g
- Saturated Fat: 2g
- Carbohydrates: 24g
- Fiber: 7g
- Sugars: 15g
- Protein: 3g

4. Greek Yogurt Parfait with Granola and Berries

Prep Time: 5 minutes
Cooking Time: 0 minutes
Serving Size: 2

Ingredients:

- 1 cup plain Greek yogurt
- ½ cup granola (look for low-sugar or homemade varieties)
- ½ cup mixed berries (strawberries, blueberries, raspberries)
- Drizzle of honey or maple syrup (optional)

Instructions:

1. In serving glasses or bowls, layer Greek yogurt, granola, and mixed berries.
2. Repeat the layers until the glasses are filled.

3. Optionally, drizzle honey or maple syrup over the top for added sweetness.

4. Serve immediately as a satisfying and nutritious dessert or snack.

Nutritional Information (per serving):

- Calories: 250

- Total Fat: 6g

- Saturated Fat: 1g

- Carbohydrates: 30g

- Fiber: 5g

- Sugars: 15g

- Protein: 20g

5. Coconut Mango Popsicles

Prep Time: 10 minutes
Freezing Time: 4 hours
Serving Size: 4

Ingredients:

- 1 ripe mango, peeled and diced

- 1 cup coconut milk (canned, full-fat)

- 2 tablespoons honey or maple syrup

- 1 teaspoon vanilla extract

Instructions:

1. In a blender, combine diced mango, coconut milk, honey or maple syrup, and vanilla extract.

2. Blend until smooth and creamy.

3. Pour the mixture into popsicle molds, leaving a little space at the top for expansion.

4. Insert popsicle sticks into each mold.

5. Freeze for at least 4 hours or until solid.

6. To release the popsicles, run the molds under warm water for a few seconds.

7. Enjoy these refreshing coconut mango popsicles on a hot day!

Nutritional Information (per serving):

- Calories: 150

- Total Fat: 8g

- Saturated Fat: 7g

- Carbohydrates: 20g

- Fiber: 2g

- Sugars: 17g

- Protein: 1g

6. Lemon Blueberry Yogurt Bark

Prep Time: 10 minutes
Freezing Time: 2 hours
Serving Size: 4

Ingredients:

- 2 cups plain Greek yogurt

- Zest and juice of 1 lemon

- 2 tablespoons honey or maple syrup

- ½ cup fresh blueberries

Instructions:

1. In a mixing bowl, combine Greek yogurt, lemon zest, lemon juice, and honey or maple syrup.

2. Line a baking sheet with parchment paper.

3. Spread the yogurt mixture evenly onto the parchment paper, about 1/4 inch thick.

4. Scatter fresh blueberries over the yogurt mixture, pressing them gently into the surface.

5. Freeze the yogurt bark for at least 2 hours or until firm.

6. Once frozen, break the bark into pieces using your hands or a knife.

7. Serve immediately as a refreshing and satisfying dessert or snack.

Nutritional Information (per serving):

- Calories: 120

- Total Fat: 0g

- Saturated Fat: 0g

- Carbohydrates: 18g

- Fiber: 1g

- Sugars: 15g

- Protein: 11g

7. Almond Butter Banana Bites

Prep Time: 10 minutes
Freezing Time: 1 hour
Serving Size: 2

Ingredients:

- 1 ripe banana, peeled and sliced into rounds

- 2 tablespoons almond butter

- Optional toppings: Unsweetened shredded coconut, chopped nuts

Instructions:

1. Spread almond butter on half of the banana slices.

2. Sandwich the almond butter-coated slices with the remaining banana slices to form "banana bites."

3. Place the banana bites on a baking sheet lined with parchment paper.

4. Optionally, sprinkle with unsweetened shredded coconut or chopped nuts for added texture and flavour.

5. Freeze the banana bites for at least 1 hour or until firm.

6. Serve these delicious and nutritious almond butter banana bites as a guilt-free dessert or snack.

Nutritional Information (per serving):

- Calories: 180

- Total Fat: 9g

- Saturated Fat: 1g

- Carbohydrates: 23g

- Fiber: 3g

- Sugars: 13g

- Protein: 5g

8. Pumpkin Spice Energy Bites

Prep Time: 10 minutes
Chilling Time: 30 minutes
Serving Size: 6

Ingredients:

- 1 cup rolled oats

- ½ cup pumpkin puree

- ¼ cup almond butter

- 2 tablespoons honey or maple syrup

- 1 teaspoon pumpkin pie spice

- ¼ cup unsweetened shredded coconut (for rolling)

Instructions:

1. In a mixing bowl, combine rolled oats, pumpkin puree, almond butter, honey or maple syrup, and pumpkin pie spice.

2. Stir until well combined and the mixture holds together.

3. Place the shredded coconut in a shallow dish.

4. Roll the oat mixture into bite-sized balls, then roll each ball in the shredded coconut to coat.

5. Place the energy bites on a plate or baking sheet lined with parchment paper.

6. Chill the energy bites in the refrigerator for at least 30 minutes before serving.

7. Enjoy these flavourful and nutritious pumpkin spice energy bites as a satisfying snack or dessert.

Nutritional Information (per serving):

- Calories: 150

- Total Fat: 6g

- Saturated Fat: 2g

- Carbohydrates: 22g

- Fiber: 3g

- Sugars: 9g

- Protein: 4g

9. Cinnamon Baked Pears

Prep Time: 10 minutes
Cooking Time: 30 minutes
Serving Size: 2

Ingredients:

- 2 ripe pears, halved and cored

- 1 tablespoon lemon juice

- 1 teaspoon ground cinnamon

- Optional: Drizzle of honey or maple syrup

Instructions:

1. Preheat the oven to 375°F (190°C).

2. Place the pear halves in a baking dish, cut side up.

3. Drizzle lemon juice over the pears to prevent browning.

4. Sprinkle ground cinnamon evenly over the pears.

5. Optionally, drizzle with honey or maple syrup for added sweetness.

6. Bake in the preheated oven for 25-30 minutes or until the pears are tender.

7. Serve warm as a comforting and nutritious dessert option.

Nutritional Information (per serving):

- Calories: 100
- Total Fat: 0g
- Saturated Fat: 0g
- Carbohydrates: 26g
- Fiber: 6g
- Sugars: 16g
- Protein: 1g

10. Chocolate Covered Strawberries

Prep Time: 15 minutes
Chilling Time: 30 minutes
Serving Size: 4

Ingredients:

- 1 cup fresh strawberries, rinsed and dried
- 2 ounces dark chocolate (70% cocoa or higher), chopped
- 1 teaspoon coconut oil
- Optional toppings: Chopped nuts, shredded coconut

Instructions:

1. Line a baking sheet with parchment paper.
2. In a heatproof bowl, combine chopped dark chocolate and coconut oil.

3. Microwave in 30-second intervals, stirring between each interval, until the chocolate is melted and smooth.

4. Holding each strawberry by the stem, dip it into the melted chocolate, coating it halfway.

5. Place the chocolate-covered strawberries on the prepared baking sheet.

6. Optionally, sprinkle with chopped nuts or shredded coconut before the chocolate sets.

7. Chill the strawberries in the refrigerator for at least 30 minutes or until the chocolate is firm.

8. Serve these elegant and decadent chocolate-covered strawberries as a delightful dessert or special treat.

Nutritional Information (per serving):

- Calories: 80

- Total Fat: 5g

- Saturated Fat: 3g

- Carbohydrates: 10g

- Fiber: 3g

- Sugars: 6g

- Protein: 1g

CHAPTER 8

SAMPLE MEAL PLAN

Day 1:

- **Breakfast:** Greek Yogurt Parfait with Granola and Berries
- **Lunch:** Colourful Salad with Grilled Chicken
- **Dinner:** Baked Apples with Cinnamon
- **Snack:** Almond Butter Banana Bites
- **Dessert:** Coconut Mango Popsicles

Day 2:

- **Breakfast:** Berry Chia Seed Pudding
- **Lunch:** Quinoa Salad with Roasted Vegetables
- **Dinner:** Lemon Blueberry Yogurt Bark
- **Snack:** Pumpkin Spice Energy Bites
- **Dessert:** Chocolate Avocado Mousse

Day 3:

- **Breakfast:** Chocolate Avocado Mousse
- **Lunch:** Turkey Wrap with Mixed Greens
- **Dinner:** Cinnamon Baked Pears
- **Snack:** Coconut Mango Popsicles
- **Dessert:** Almond Butter Banana Bites

Day 4:

- **Breakfast:** Baked Apples with Cinnamon
- **Lunch:** Lentil Soup with Whole Grain Bread
- **Dinner:** Chocolate Covered Strawberries
- **Snack:** Lemon Blueberry Yogurt Bark
- **Dessert:** Berry Chia Seed Pudding

Day 5:

- **Breakfast:** Berry Chia Seed Pudding
- **Lunch:** Greek Salad with Grilled Shrimp
- **Dinner:** Coconut Mango Popsicles
- **Snack:** Pumpkin Spice Energy Bites
- **Dessert:** Greek Yogurt Parfait with Granola and Berries

Day 6:

- **Breakfast:** Lemon Blueberry Yogurt Bark
- **Lunch:** Chickpea Salad with Lemon Tahini Dressing
- **Dinner:** Greek Yogurt Parfait with Granola and Berries
- **Snack:** Chocolate Covered Strawberries
- **Dessert:** Cinnamon Baked Pears

Day 7:

- **Breakfast:** Pumpkin Spice Energy Bites
- **Lunch:** Quinoa Salad with Roasted Vegetables
- **Dinner:** Almond Butter Banana Bites
- **Snack:** Coconut Mango Popsicles
- **Dessert:** Lemon Blueberry Yogurt Bark

Day 8:

- **Breakfast:** Chocolate Avocado Mousse
- **Lunch:** Colourful Salad with Grilled Chicken
- **Dinner:** Baked Apples with Cinnamon
- **Snack:** Berry Chia Seed Pudding
- **Dessert:** Pumpkin Spice Energy Bites

Day 9:

- **Breakfast:** Baked Apples with Cinnamon
- **Lunch:** Lentil Soup with Whole Grain Bread
- **Dinner:** Chocolate Covered Strawberries
- **Snack:** Coconut Mango Popsicles
- **Dessert:** Greek Yogurt Parfait with Granola and Berries

Day 10:

- **Breakfast:** Lemon Blueberry Yogurt Bark
- **Lunch:** Greek Salad with Grilled Shrimp

- **Dinner:** Coconut Mango Popsicles

- **Snack:** Almond Butter Banana Bites

- **Dessert:** Chocolate Avocado Mousse

Day 11:

- **Breakfast:** Berry Chia Seed Pudding

- **Lunch:** Chickpea Salad with Lemon Tahini Dressing

- **Dinner:** Greek Yogurt Parfait with Granola and Berries

- **Snack:** Chocolate Covered Strawberries

- **Dessert:** Baked Apples with Cinnamon

Day 12:

- **Breakfast:** Pumpkin Spice Energy Bites

- **Lunch:** Quinoa Salad with Roasted Vegetables

- **Dinner:** Almond Butter Banana Bites

- **Snack:** Coconut Mango Popsicles

- **Dessert:** Lemon Blueberry Yogurt Bark

Day 13:

- **Breakfast:** Chocolate Avocado Mousse

- **Lunch:** Colourful Salad with Grilled Chicken

- **Dinner:** Coconut Mango Popsicles

- **Snack:** Berry Chia Seed Pudding

- **Dessert:** Pumpkin Spice Energy Bites

Day 14:

- **Breakfast:** Baked Apples with Cinnamon
- **Lunch:** Lentil Soup with Whole Grain Bread
- **Dinner:** Chocolate Covered Strawberries
- **Snack:** Greek Yogurt Parfait with Granola and Berries
- **Dessert:** Almond Butter Banana Bites

Day 15:

- **Breakfast:** Lemon Blueberry Yogurt Bark
- **Lunch:** Greek Salad with Grilled Shrimp
- **Dinner:** Greek Yogurt Parfait with Granola and Berries
- **Snack:** Coconut Mango Popsicles
- **Dessert:** Chocolate Avocado Mousse

Day 16:

- **Breakfast:** Berry Chia Seed Pudding
- **Lunch:** Chickpea Salad with Lemon Tahini Dressing
- **Dinner:** Cinnamon Baked Pears
- **Snack:** Pumpkin Spice Energy Bites
- **Dessert:** Baked Apples with Cinnamon

Day 17:

- **Breakfast:** Pumpkin Spice Energy Bites
- **Lunch:** Quinoa Salad with Roasted Vegetables
- **Dinner:** Lemon Blueberry Yogurt Bark
- **Snack:** Almond Butter Banana Bites
- **Dessert:** Coconut Mango Popsicles

Day 18:

- **Breakfast:** Chocolate Avocado Mousse
- **Lunch:** Colourful Salad with Grilled Chicken
- **Dinner:** Chocolate Covered Strawberries
- **Snack:** Greek Yogurt Parfait with Granola and Berries
- **Dessert:** Berry Chia Seed Pudding

Day 19:

- **Breakfast:** Baked Apples with Cinnamon
- **Lunch:** Lentil Soup with Whole Grain Bread
- **Dinner:** Almond Butter Banana Bites
- **Snack:** Lemon Blueberry Yogurt Bark
- **Dessert:** Pumpkin Spice Energy Bites

Day 20:

- **Breakfast:** Lemon Blueberry Yogurt Bark
- **Lunch:** Greek Salad with Grilled Shrimp

- **Dinner:** Coconut Mango Popsicles

- **Snack:** Chocolate Avocado Mousse

- **Dessert:** Greek Yogurt Parfait with Granola and Berries

Day 21:

- **Breakfast:** Berry Chia Seed Pudding

- **Lunch:** Chickpea Salad with Lemon Tahini Dressing

- **Dinner:** Chocolate Avocado Mousse

- **Snack:** Coconut Mango Popsicles

- **Dessert:** Baked Apples with Cinnamon

Day 22:

- **Breakfast:** Pumpkin Spice Energy Bites

- **Lunch:** Quinoa Salad with Roasted Vegetables

- **Dinner:** Almond Butter Banana Bites

- **Snack:** Lemon Blueberry Yogurt Bark

- **Dessert:** Chocolate Covered Strawberries

Day 23:

- **Breakfast:** Chocolate Avocado Mousse

- **Lunch:** Colourful Salad with Grilled Chicken

- **Dinner:** Coconut Mango Popsicles

- **Snack:** Greek Yogurt Parfait with Granola and Berries

- **Dessert:** Berry Chia Seed Pudding

Day 24:

- **Breakfast:** Baked Apples with Cinnamon

- **Lunch:** Lentil Soup with Whole Grain Bread

- **Dinner:** Lemon Blueberry Yogurt Bark

- **Snack:** Pumpkin Spice Energy Bites

- **Dessert:** Greek Yogurt Parfait with Granola and Berries

Day 25:

- **Breakfast:** Lemon Blueberry Yogurt Bark

- **Lunch:** Greek Salad with Grilled Shrimp

- **Dinner:** Greek Yogurt Parfait with Granola and Berries

- **Snack:** Coconut Mango Popsicles

- **Dessert:** Almond Butter Banana Bites

Day 26:

- **Breakfast:** Berry Chia Seed Pudding

- **Lunch:** Chickpea Salad with Lemon Tahini Dressing

- **Dinner:** Baked Apples with Cinnamon

- **Snack:** Chocolate Covered Strawberries

- **Dessert:** Pumpkin Spice Energy Bites

Day 27:

- **Breakfast:** Pumpkin Spice Energy Bites
- **Lunch:** Quinoa Salad with Roasted Vegetables
- **Dinner:** Chocolate Avocado Mousse
- **Snack:** Lemon Blueberry Yogurt Bark
- **Dessert:** Coconut Mango Popsicles

Day 28:

- **Breakfast:** Chocolate Avocado Mousse
- **Lunch:** Colourful Salad with Grilled Chicken
- **Dinner:** Almond Butter Banana Bites
- **Snack:** Greek Yogurt Parfait with Granola and Berries
- **Dessert:** Baked Apples with Cinnamon

Day 29:

- **Breakfast:** Baked Apples with Cinnamon
- **Lunch:** Lentil Soup with Whole Grain Bread
- **Dinner:** Lemon Blueberry Yogurt Bark
- **Snack:** Pumpkin Spice Energy Bites
- **Dessert:** Berry Chia Seed Pudding

Day 30:

- **Breakfast:** Lemon Blueberry Yogurt Bark
- **Lunch:** Greek Salad with Grilled Shrimp

- **Dinner:** Greek Yogurt Parfait with Granola and Berries

- **Snack:** Coconut Mango Popsicles

- **Dessert:** Chocolate Covered Strawberries

CHAPTER 9

CONCLUSION

In the journey towards health and wellness, embarking on the Metabolic Confusion Diet presents both challenges and opportunities for transformation. As we conclude our exploration of this dietary approach, it's important to reflect on the progress made, acknowledge the obstacles faced, and embrace the potential for positive change. Through 30 days of mindful eating, we've delved into a diverse array of nutritious recipes, from vibrant salads to indulgent desserts, each designed to nourish both body and soul.

For many of us, the decision to adopt a new dietary regimen stem from a deep desire for improved health, increased energy, and a greater sense of well-being. Whether you're striving to shed a few pounds, boost your metabolism, or simply cultivate healthier eating habits, the Metabolic Confusion Diet offers a roadmap to achieving your wellness goals. By strategically alternating between different types of foods and meal compositions, this approach aims to keep your metabolism guessing, ultimately promoting fat loss, muscle retention, and overall metabolic balance.

Yet, amidst the promise of transformation, we cannot overlook the inevitable challenges that accompany any dietary change. From battling cravings to navigating social situations, staying committed to your health journey requires dedication, resilience, and a steadfast belief in your ability to succeed. It's important to remember that setbacks are a natural part of the process, and each stumble serves as an opportunity to learn, grow, and recalibrate your approach. As you journey through the ups and downs of the Metabolic Confusion Diet, know that you are not alone. Countless individuals, just like you, are striving to create healthier, happier lives, one meal at a time.

In closing, I want to extend my deepest appreciation to each and every one of you who has joined me on this culinary adventure. Your commitment to prioritizing your health and wellness is both commendable and inspiring. As we bid farewell to this chapter, let us carry forward the lessons learned, the habits formed, and the newfound sense of empowerment that comes from nourishing our bodies with intention and purpose.

Remember, the journey towards optimal health is not a sprint but a marathon—a journey of self-discovery, resilience, and unwavering determination. So, as you continue along your path, may you find solace in the knowledge that every step forward, no matter how small, brings you closer to the vibrant, radiant life you deserve.

In the words of Ralph Waldo Emerson, "The first wealth is health." As we embrace the endless possibilities that lie ahead, let us remain steadfast in our pursuit of health, happiness, and vitality. Together, we can achieve anything we set our minds to.

Here's to your continued success, growth, and well-being. Cheers to a life lived with purpose, passion, and unwavering commitment to self-care. The best is yet to come!

www.ingramcontent.com/pod-product-compliance
Lightning Source LLC
Chambersburg PA
CBHW050820260726
48660CB00004B/1536